Pathways in Prosthetic Joint Infection

T0177744

Pathways in Prosthetic Joint Infection

Mr Umraz Khan
Mr Graeme Perks
Mr Rhidian Morgan-Jones
Mr Peter James
Mr Colin Esler
Mr Vince Smyth
Dr Vanya Gant

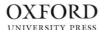

OXFORD
UNIVERSITY PRESS

Great Clarendon Street, Oxford, OX2 6DP,
United Kingdom

Oxford University Press is a department of the University of Oxford.
It furthers the University's objective of excellence in research, scholarship,
and education by publishing worldwide. Oxford is a registered trade mark of
Oxford University Press in the UK and in certain other countries

First Edition published in 2018

Impression: 1

Published in the United States of America by Oxford University Press
198 Madison Avenue, New York, NY 10016, United States of America

British Library Cataloguing in Publication Data

Data available

Library of Congress Control Number: 2018941861

ISBN 978–0–19–879188–1

Printed in Great Britain by
Ashford Colour Press Ltd, Gosport, Hampshire

Endorsements

Periprosthetic joint infection is one of the most devastating and costly outcomes following knee arthroplasty surgery. It is best managed by a multidisciplinary team to eradicate the infection successfully and maximize the chance of the patient having a knee that has satisfactory function and minimal pain. Periprosthetic infection is an independent predictor of mortality, and resistant organisms threaten the viability of arthroplasty surgery. This publication summarizes our current knowledge and should assist clinicians and commissioners to develop management strategies and services that patients deserve.

President of the British Association for Surgery of the Knee

The Vascular Society is glad to see a comprehensive multidisciplinary approach to the complex issue of infection in prosthetic materials. In this era of increasingly complex interventions and antibiotic-resistant organisms, the principles of eradication, optimization, and reconstruction are applicable to any speciality using non-autologous elements. These should form part of the understanding of any surgeon who deals with such clinical scenarios.

Vascular Society for Great Britain and Ireland

The diagnosis of a prosthetic joint infection (PJI) is devastating and challenging, and both surgeon and patient fear it. Fortunately it remains an uncommon occurrence. The ethos of getting it right first time (GIRFT) demands that this risk remains uncommon and that efficacious pathways exist for the management of cases of PJI. The publication of this book is a timely one as it crystallizes both GIRFT and the spirit of collaborative care, both of which aim to improve outcomes. It is anticipated that the need for the pathways described within this book would be of clinical use as the demand for arthroplasty as well as revision arthroplasty increases globally. The book is well-written by experts, bringing together a collective experience in this field. The authors have reviewed the current literature and have made recommendations based upon that as well as their individual experience. As the national lead of GIRFT I would support this book to all clinicians caring for patients who develop PJI.

Professor Tim Briggs CBE
Professor of Orthopaedic Surgery
National Lead GIRFT
2018

Foreword from the Royal College of Surgeons

I remember so clearly the first time I realized that a patient on whom I had operated had developed a deep joint infection. I remember his name, the microbiological findings, his face when I explained to him the consequences, and the months of our subsequent interactions. Probably the most difficult aspect was that then I had no experience, many others were in denial, and there was no clear guidance, cohesive and well-researched pathway or networks from whom to ask for help.

The British Association of Plastic, Reconstructive and Aesthetic Surgeons, the British Orthopaedic Association, The Vascular Society and Microbiology have, in this publication, brought together the knowledge and work of experts in the science and art of management of these very difficult cases. A clear document that guides us through the diagnosis and management, and the literature to back it up, is most welcome. Standardized evidence-based management is likely to give the best chance of the patient benefitting once they have been unfortunate enough to develop these complications.

Prompt diagnosis, honesty, and expertise must be the watch words for those clinicians faced with the care of these patients. In difficult cases such as these we need all the help we can get, and an authoritative work such as this is a critical element of that help.

Clare Marx
Former President, Royal College of Surgeons of England
December 2016

Foreword from the British Association of Plastic, Reconstructive and Aesthetic Surgeons

Prosthetic joint infection is a major complication, leads to functional problems, and may need revisional surgery. In the past a multidisciplinary team approach to managing such infections was sometimes lacking, compromising a patient's chance of achieving a good final outcome. Now, the collaboration between specialties that has led to the pathways described will improve patients' care significantly and will help improve outcomes.

The pathways here encompass not only surgical treatment when an infection is established but also, and most importantly, risk factors and prevention. They are an essential part of modern care, and BAPRAS is proud to be part of the authorship.

David Ward
President BAPRAS
January 2017

Contents

Authors

Mr Umraz Khan
Chairman of the Working Group and
BAPRAS Lead & Consultant Plastic
Surgeon, North Bristol NHS Trust,
Bristol, UK

Mr Graeme Perks
Head of the Department of Plastic,
Reconstructive and Burns Surgery,
Nottingham University Hospitals NHS
Trust, Nottingham, UK

Mr Rhidian Morgan-Jones
Consultant Orthopaedic Surgeon &
Honorary Lecturer, University Hospital of
Wales, Cardiff, UK

Mr Peter James
Consultant Hip and Knee Surgeon,
Nottingham University Hospital,
Nottingham, UK

Mr Colin Esler
Consultant & Honorary Senior Lecturer
in Trauma and Orthopaedic Surgery,
Leicester General Hospital, Leicester, UK

Mr Vince Smyth
Consultant Vascular and Endovascular
Surgeon, Manchester Royal Infirmary,
Manchester, UK

Dr Vanya Gant
Clinical Director for Infection and
Consultant Microbiologist, University
College London, London, UK

Chapter 1

Introduction

Elective orthopaedic surgery has become commonplace, comprising approximately 25% of all medical activity in the National Health Service (NHS). This growth has been attributed to the success of the procedures in alleviating symptoms as well as advances in implant technology driven by industry. It has also been acknowledged, however, that revisional surgery is on the increase and that some procedures have a low level of clinical evidence of effectiveness. This has prompted the publication of critical analysis of practice in arthroplasty surgery in the form of a document 'Getting it Right First Time' (GIRFT, 2015), which emphasizes the importance of thoroughness of preoperative analysis.

The battle to reduce surgical site infection continues with attention to theatre protocol and antibiotic prophylaxis. Prosthetic joint infection (PJI) is a feared complication of arthroplasty and, although the incidence has been reduced, it is not zero. The threat of amputation proximal to the affected joint remains a significant risk to those affected by PJI, but to others there may be significant morbidity and even mortality from sepsis. Prevention must remain the aim of all practitioners. However, when PJI occurs there remains inconsistency in the pathways available to offer patients. Furthermore, it has been suggested that suffering a PJI increases 1-year mortality (Zmistowski et al., 2013).

There are reported to be over 3500 publications on PJI (Gehrke and Parvizi, 2013). These cover topics such as risk factors associated with increased surgical site infection (SSI)/PJI, perioperative skin preparation, perioperative antibiotics, operative environment, blood conservation, prosthesis selection, diagnosis of PJI, wound management, spacers, irrigation and debridement, antibiotic treatment and timing of reimplantation, one-stage versus two-stage exchange arthroplasty, oral antibiotic therapy, and prevention of late PJI. This document aims to distil contemporary literature by expert practitioners to provide an evidence base for safe and effective practice.

Defining periprosthetic joint infection

Based on the proposed criteria, a definite diagnosis of PJI (Parvizi, 2014) can be made when the following conditions are met:

A sinus tract communicating with the prosthesis; or

A pathogen is isolated by culture from two separate tissue or fluid samples obtained from the affected prosthetic joint; or

Four of the following six criteria exist:

Elevated serum erythrocyte sedimentation rate (ESR>30 mm/h) or serum C-reactive protein concentration (CRP>10 mg/L) (Della Vale et al., 2007; Toms et al., 2006).

Elevated synovial white blood cell count (WCC>1100 cells/µL in chronic cases (Ahlberg et al., 1978), WCC>27,800 cells/µL in acute cases) (Bedair et al., 2011).

Elevated synovial neutrophil percentage (PMN>64%) (Ghanem et al., 2008).

Presence of purulence in the affected joint.

Isolation of a microorganism in one culture of periprosthetic tissue or fluid.

Greater than five neutrophils per high-power field in five high-power fields observed from histological analysis of periprosthetic tissue at 400 times magnification.

However, it should be noted that PJI may be present even if fewer than four of these criteria are met (Parvizi, 2014).

Classification of surgical site infections

Definitions of SSIs are based on those published by the Centers for Disease Control (CDC), and are classified as incisional (superficial or deep) or organ/space infection.

Superficial incisional infection: this is defined as an SSI that occurs within 30 days of surgery and involves only the skin or subcutaneous tissue of the incision, and meets at least one of the following criteria:

Criterion 1: Purulent drainage from the superficial incision.

Criterion 2: The superficial incision yields organisms from the culture of aseptically aspirated fluid or tissue, or from a swab, and pus cells are present.

Criterion 3: At least two of the following symptoms and signs:

- pain or tenderness
- localized swelling
- redness
- heat and
  a. the superficial incision is deliberately opened by a surgeon to manage the infection, unless the incision is culture-negative or
  b. the clinician diagnoses a superficial incisional infection.

Note: stitch abscesses are defined as minimal inflammation and discharge confined to the points of suture penetration, and localized infection around a stab wound. They are not classified as SSIs.

Deep incisional infection: this is defined as an SSI involving the deep tissues (i.e. fascial and muscle layers) that occurs within 30 days of surgery if no implant is in place, or within 1 year if an implant is in place and the infection appears to be related to the surgical procedure. It meets at least one of the following criteria:

Criterion 1: Purulent drainage from the deep incision but not from the organ/space component of the surgical site.

Criterion 2: The deep incision yields organisms from the culture of aseptically aspirated fluid or tissue, or from a swab, and pus cells are present.

Criterion 3: A deep incision that spontaneously dehisces or is deliberately opened by a surgeon when the patient has at least one of the following symptoms or signs (unless the incision is culture-negative):

- fever (>38°C)
- localized pain or tenderness.

Criterion 4: An abscess or other evidence of infection involving the deep incision that is found by direct examination during reoperation or by histopathological or radiological examination.

Criterion 5: Diagnosis of a deep incisional SSI by an attending clinician. Note: An infection involving both superficial and deep incision is classified as deep incisional SSI unless there are different organisms present at each site.

Organ/space infection: this is defined as an SSI involving any part of the anatomy (i.e. organ/space) other than the incision, opened or manipulated during the surgical procedure, that occurs within 30 days of surgery if no implant is in place, or within 1 year if an implant is in place and the infection appears to be related to the surgical procedure. It meets at least one of the following criteria:

Criterion 1: Purulent drainage from a drain that is placed through a stab wound into the organ/space.

Criterion 2: The organ/space yields organisms from the culture of aseptically aspirated fluid or tissue, or from a swab, and pus cells are present.

Criterion 3: An abscess or other evidence of infection involving the organ/space that is found by direct examination, during reoperation, or by histopathological or radiological examination.

Criterion 4: Diagnosis of an organ/space infection by an attending clinician.

Note: occasionally an organ/space infection drains through the incision. Such infection generally does not require reoperation and is considered to be a complication of the incision, and is therefore classified as a deep incisional infection.

Incidence of prosthetic joint infection in total knee replacement

Joint replacement surgery is the most common procedure performed in most orthopaedic institutions. In England and Wales alone more than 175,000 hip and knee replacements were conducted in 2012 (National Joint Registry). There has been a steady increase in the demand for total knee arthroplasty (TKR) and total hip arthroplasty (THR) as a result of the aging population and the outstanding long-term results. These can be attributed to technological advancements in prosthetic design, instrumentation, and surgical technique (Johanson et al., 1999). Joint replacement surgery has proven to be the most cost-effective procedure for patients with end-stage joint disease (Callahan et al., 1998). Estimated projections for primary and revision hip and knee arthroplasty in the USA by 2030 show truly extraordinary increases: a 673% increase in primary TKR and a 174% increase in primary THR; a 601% increase in revision TKR and 137% increase in revision THR (Kurtz et al., 2009). As the 'at-risk' population expands dramatically, so too will the burden of revision, and the incidence and prevalence of periprosthetic joint infection will increase over time (Kurtz et al., 2007; 2008). PJI is rare following hip and knee arthroplasty; however, infection is the commonest mode of early failure of TKR (Sharkey et al., 2002).

How do we quantify prosthetic joint infection?

There are four areas where the incidence of PJI can be quantified: personal, institutional, published, and national.

1. Personal

Sir John Charnley is quoted as saying 'Nothing destroys the reputation of a surgeon like infection' and this is surely true. However, surgeons may have the habit of overlooking or denying their infections. It is often said that infection is easier to diagnose in other surgeons' arthroplasty operations than one's own. The authors therefore urge surgeons to keep their own database of PJIs ('an honesty table') so that the operating surgeon can reflect on each case and look for any factors that can be improved or changed in future.

2. Institutional

All hospitals performing arthroplasty surgery should have a clear record of their institutional PJI rates. The Hospital for Special Surgery (HSS) in New York in 2015 (www.hss.edu) states in their promotional literature that 'the risk of infection from total knee replacement is less than 1%'. Closer to home, the Royal National Orthopaedic Hospital, Stanmore quotes a 0.2% primary PJI rate (GIRFT, 2015). In Wales, the All-Wales Orthopaedic Surgical Site Infection Surveillance puts University Hospital Llandough combined deep and superficial knee arthroplasty infection rate at 2.2% (85% being superficial) in 2010 (www.wales.nhs.uk).

3. National

On a national level, with the largest denominator arthroplasties, one would hope to find an accurate incidence of PJI. The American Academy of Orthopaedic Surgeons (http://www.aaos.org) states on its website (2015) that the 'realistic risk of infection with current surgical techniques and antibiotic regimens is about 0.5%'; the British Orthopaedic Association (BOA) makes no such statements. Looking at the Medicare database (http://www.medicare.gov), however, reveals the incidence of infected TKR in the USA to be 0.6–1.9% in 2010. In Wales, the All-Wales 30-day SSI (deep and superficial) data in 2007 (www.wales.nhs.uk) shows a rate of hip arthroplasty infection of 2.3% and infected knee arthroplasty of 3.2%. Combined SSI, deep and superficial, using CDC definitions for total primary knee prosthesis is widely accepted at around 3% (Lopez-Contreras et al., 2012).

Possibly the most accurate rates of PJI will come from National Joint Registries (NJRs). The UK has the largest registry in the world, with over 1 million arthroplasties enrolled. The UK NJR reports that 23% of all revision knees are undertaken for infection, with an annual incidence of deep infection of 1.4% (http://www.njrcentre. org.uk).

4. Published

Infection, although uncommon, is the most serious complication, occurring in 0.8–1.9% of knee arthroplasties and 0.3–1.7% of hip arthroplasties (Del Pozo and Patel, 2009), but this may represent an underestimate (Jamsen et al., 2009). In one series, 19% of TKRs were revised for infection and the overall incidence of infection after revision TKR was 9.2% (Mortazavi et al., 2010). The published incidence of PJI varies between joints and procedures. In 2003, Strengel et al. reported a lower incidence in hip arthroplasty (primary 0.5–1%, revision 1–4%) than knee arthroplasty (primary 1–1.5%, revision 2–4%) whilst the highest rates were seen in shoulder arthroplasty (total shoulder 1.5%, reversed total shoulder 6–10%). Revision TKR in all series has a higher infection rate than primary TKR, with rates of 4.2–5.8% reported (Blom et al., 2004; Khatod et al., 2008). The cumulative incidence of PJI increases with time after implantation, almost trebling in one series from 0.5% at year 1 to 0.8% at year 5 and 1.4% 10 years after arthroplasty (Tsaras et al., 2012).

It thus seems that the incidence of PJI varies depending upon how these data are gathered.

The burden of prosthetic joint infection

Infection still remains one of the major complications leading to functional impairment and, at worst, revision surgery, with an associated mortality of 2.7–18% (Powers et al., 1990; Ahlberg et al., 1978). Surgeons must also be cognisant of the systemic impact of periprosthetic joint infection and its major influence on fatal outcome in patients (Zmistowski et al., 2013). Infected cases lead to increased patient morbidity, extensive medical and surgical treatment, and pose a significant financial burden to hospital trusts. It has been calculated in the USA that an infected TKR produces increased length of hospitalization, readmissions, and associated medical and surgical care equating to a mean annual cost of $116,383 as opposed to $28,249 when compared to a matched group (Kapadia et al., 2014). The predicted rise in revision cases even with a baseline infection rate of 1% would equate to thousands of extra cases of infection per year, which will have a significant impact on healthcare provision in the NHS.

Conclusion

The trend worldwide is for the total number of arthroplasties to increase; as this occurs the total revision burden will also increase and it is inevitable that there will be an increase in PJI. Current reported deep infection rates in the UK are 1.4% for TKR but this will involve 23% of all revision TKR. PJI leads to increased patient morbidity and mortality and a significant increase in healthcare costs.

References

Ahlberg A, Carlsson AS, Lindgren L. Hematogenous infection in total joint replacement. *Clin Orthop Relat Res.* 1978;137:69–75.

Bedair H, Ting N, Parvizi J, et al. The Mark Coventry Award: Diagnosis of early post-operative TKA infection using synovial fluid analysis. *Clin Orthop Relat Res.* 2011;469(1):34–40.

Blom AW, Brown J, Taylor AH, Pattison G, Whitehouse S, Bannister GC. Infection after total knee arthroplasty. *J Bone Joint Surg Br.* 2004;86(5):688–91.

Callahan CM, Drake BG, Heck DA, Dittus RS. Patient outcomes following tricompartmental total knee replacement. *JAMA.* 1998;271(17):257–65.

Della Vale CJ, Sporer SM, Jacobs JJ, Berger RA, Rosenberg AG, Paprosky WG. Pre-operative testing for sepsis before revision total knee arthroplasty. *J Arthroplasty.* 2007;22(6):90–3.

Del Pozo P, Patel R. Clinical practice. Infection associated with prosthetic joints. *N Engl J Med.* 2009;361(8):787–94.

Gehrke T, Parvizi J. (2013). *Proceedings of the International Consensus meeting on Peri-Prosthetic Joint Infection.* https://www.efort.org/wp-content/uploads/2013/10/Philadelphia_Consensus.pdf

Ghanem E, Parvizi J, Burnett RS, et al. Cell count and differential of aspirated fluid in the diagnosis of infection at the site of total knee arthroplasty. *J Bone Joint Surg Am.* 2008;90(8):1637–43.

GIRFT (2015). www.gettingitrightfirsttime.com

Jämsen E, Huotari K, Huhtala H, Nevalainen J, Konttinen YT. Low rate of infected knee replacements in a nationwide series—is it an underestimate? *Acta Orthop.* 2009;80(2):205–12.

Johanson N, Michael S, Burrows B. Results of revision knee replacement with standard, modular, and constrained devices. In: Lotke PA, Garino JP (eds). *Revision Total Knee Arthroplasty.* Philadelphia: LippincottRaven, 1999: pp. 355–70.

Kapadia BH, McElroy MJ, Issa K, Johnson AJ, Bozic KJ, Mont MA. The economic impact of periprosthetic infections following total knee arthroplasty at a specialized tertiary-care center. *J Arthroplasty.* 2014;29(5):929–32.

Khatod M, Inacio M, Paxton EW, et al. Knee replacement: epidemiology, outcomes, and trends in Southern California: 17,080 replacements from 1995 through 2004. *Acta Orthop.* 2008;79(6):812–19.

Kurtz SM, Ong KL, Schmier J, et al. Future clinical and economic impact of revision total hip and knee arthroplasty. *J Bone Joint Surg Am.* 2007;89 (Suppl. 3):144–51.

Kurtz SM, Lau E, Schmier J, Ong KL, Zhao K, Parvizi J. Infection burden for hip and knee arthroplasty in the United States. *J Arthroplasty.* 2008;23(7):984–91.

Kurtz SM, Ong KL, Schmier J, Zhao K, Mowat F, Lau E. Primary and revision arthroplasty surgery case-loads in the United States from 1990 to 2004. *J Arthroplasty.* 2009;24(2):195–203.

López-Contreras J, Limón E, Matas L, et al. VINCat Program. Epidemiology of surgical site infections after total hip and knee joint replacement during 2007–2009: a report from the VINCat Program. *Enferm Infecc Microbiol Clin.* 2012;30 (Suppl. 3):26–32.

Mortazavi SMJ, Schwartzenberger J, Austin MS, Purtill JJ, Parvizi J. Revision total knee arthroplasty infection. Incidence and predictors. *Clin Orthop Relat Res.* 2010;468:2052–9.

Parvizi J. A new definition for periprosthetic joint infection. *AAOS Now.* 2014;8(8):1–7.

Powers KA, Terpenning MS, Voice RA, Kauffman C. Prosthetic joint infections in the elderly. *Am J Med.* 1990;88(5N):9N–13N.

Sharkey PF, Hozack WJ, Rothman RH, Shastri S, Jacoby SM. Insall Award paper. Why are total knee arthroplasties failing today? *Clin Orthop Rel Res.* 2002;404:7–13.

Strengel D, Bauwens K, Seifert J, Ekkernkamp A. Perioperative Antibiotikaprophylaxe bei aseptischen Knochen- und Gelenkeingriffen. *Operat Orthop Traumatol.* 2003;15:101–12.

6

Toms AD, Davidson D, Masri BA, Duncan CP. The management of periprosthetic infection in total joint arthroplasty. *J Bone Joint Surg Br.* 2006;88B(2):149–55.

Tsaras G, Osmon DR, Mabry T, et al. Incidence, secular trends, and outcomes of prosthetic joint infection: a population-based study, olmsted county, Minnesota, 1969–2007. *Infect Control Hosp Epidemiol.* 2012;33(12):1207–12.

Zmistowski B, Karam JA, Durinka JB, Casper DS, Parvizi J. Periprosthetic joint infection increases the risk of one-year mortality. *J Bone Joint Surg Am.* 2013;95(24):2177–84.

Chapter 2

Assessing risk of prosthetic joint infection

High-risk patients

1. Age
2. Skin colour
3. Extracellular matrix
4. Cellular turnover
5. Diabetes
6. Obesity
7. Rheumatoid arthritis
8. Previous periarticular fractures
9. Skin disorders.

These are all independent high-risk factors for prosthetic joint infection (PJI) and require individual and prior planning to ensure that the risk posed to successful arthroplasty is minimized. Patients with a number of these risk factors are best seen in a specialist clinic (Rodriguez-Merchan, 2012; Santaguida et al., 2008). It is unknown whether these risk factors are summative

Age

There are changes to the human skin that occur as a result of both intrinsic and extrinsic factors. The skin surface changes intrinsically because of changes relating to usage of internal structures that are bound by the skin. The hands and feet, as well as the articulating joints, are such areas of the body. The lines or creases become exaggerated and deepen. This is termed chronological aging without external sun damage. With sun exposure extrinsic aging ensues. The skin wrinkles with altered pigmentation, loss of elasticity with capillary fragility leading to 'age spots'.

Skin colour

The pigments of red, yellow, blue, and brown contribute to skin colour. Melanin, flavins, and haemoglobin in various states of oxygenation are responsible for the colour. Older skin thus looks different to younger skin. This skin colour is affected in smokers, in whom the elastin is weaker.

While hyperpigmentation is most often associated with skin aging, hypopigmentation is caused by a reduction in the number of melanocytes (there is a decline of 6–8% per decade after age 30). This not only leads to a reduction in melanin (hypopigmentation), but it also accounts for a diminished protective capacity against ultraviolet (UV) exposure. Along with the decline in melanocytes, there is a reduction in both the number and functionality of the other dendritic cells of the epidermis (the Langerhans cells), which creates a lowered immune response for aged skin.

Extracellular matrix

As well as the surface (epidermal) changes the most striking change with age is in the dermis. The dermis reduces in thickness by up to 80%. The cellular basis of this lies in the dermal fibroblasts. The fibroblasts are responsible for the production of components of the extracellular matrix (ECM), especially glycosylaminoglycans (GAGs) and collagen. Fibroblasts produce fewer ECM components, resulting in a much less robust dermis and thus fragile skin. The equilibrium of biosynthesis and degradation is normally optimally balanced in young skin. The enzymes responsible for breakdown of collagen and elastin are activated by UV light. Thus the cumulative effect of sun exposure with time leads to more degradation. This, coupled with reduced GAG production, explains why older skin is more fragile.

There is less ground substance as we age, and the distribution of GAGs, such as hyaluronic acid, changes as well. This loss is most likely the cause of dehydration and loss of turgidity, which contributes to altered elasticity in aging skin.

In addition to dehydration in the dermis, studies have indicated a reduction in the moisture content of the epidermal stratum corneum, which is most likely because of a reduction in stratum corneum lipid content, resulting in less ability to bind and retain water. The result is the appearance of fine lines and scales. Fortunately, application of moisturizers and the regular use of exfoliants (in particular, exfoliants containing lactic acid) can alleviate this problem.

Cellular turnover

With age the cell turnover rate slows from 30% to 50%, thus in young adults the stratum corneum transit time is as quick as 20 days, whereas in older adults it is up to 30 days.

This prolonged stratum corneum replacement rate also coincides with a subsequent slowing of the wound healing process that is typical in older people. The slowdown in the cell cycle is combined with a less-than-efficient desquamation process, and it accounts for the characteristic dull, rough skin surface seen in maturing skin.

The human skin is thus more vulnerable and fragile, with a less predictable healing process when it ages.

It seems that age-related skin changes implicates greater age with greater vulnerability (D'Apuzzo et al., 2014). Paradoxically, those having arthroplasty under the age of 50 are at a higher risk of PJI. This often relates to the fact that younger patients will be undergoing joint replacement because of previous trauma (Meehan et al., 2014).

Diabetes

Diabetes is also seen as an independent risk factor for PJI (Jamsen et al., 2012). There is some evidence to suggest that glycaemic control prior to arthroplasty must be strictly controlled and that glycated haemoglobin be measured to assure that this is the case prior to surgery (Hwang et al., 2015).

Obesity

Obesity appears to be another independent patient-related risk factor associated with a higher incidence of PJI. The exact body mass index (BMI) that represents a threshold is unknown. However, those classified as morbidly obese with a BMI greater than 35 should be approached with caution (Font-Vizcarra et al., 2011). Obese patients will of course have greater loads across the joints of the lower limbs and have been found to have more patellofemoral disease (Stern and Insall, 1990).

Rheumatoid arthritis

Using a systematic analysis of 40 studies, Ravi et al. concluded that rheumatoid arthritis (RA) confers an increased risk in both total hip arthroplasty (THA) and total knee replacement (TKR). THA in RA is associated with a higher dislocation rate and TKR in RA with PJI (Ravi et al., 2012). This risk appears to be extra to the fact that these patients are often on medications that adversely affect wound healing. When compared with those undergoing arthroplasty for osteoarthritis those with RA have a higher incidence of PJI by a factor of 1.6 (Scharma et al., 2010). Patients with RA are generally younger than those with osteoarthritis and females predominate.

Previous periarticular fractures

Open reduction and internal fixation of fractures around the knee joint has been found to confer a higher risk of developing a PJI (Suzuki et al., 2011). The rate of PJI is increased to over 6% (Papadopoulos et al., 2002; Roffi and Merritt, 1990). The reason for this increased risk is as a result of loss of skin vascular perforators, increased scar tissue, which lacks pliability and is associated with subclinical infection. Previous tibial plateau fractures are particularly associated with a higher complication rate (Weiss et al., 2003).

Skin disorders

Psoriasis affects 1.5% of adults in the UK, whereas eczema is ten times more common. The incidence reduces in the elderly population. Both skin conditions confer an increased risk of PJI, likely due to far denser bacterial colonization of inflamed skin (Menon and Wroblewski, 1983).

References

D'Apuzzo MR, Pao AW, Novicoff WM, Browne JA. Age as an independent risk factor for postoperative morbidity and mortality after joint arthroplasty in patients 90 years of age or older. *J Arthroplasty*. 2014;29(3):477–80.

Font-Vizcarra L, Tornero E, Bori G, Bosch J, Mensa J, Soriano A. Relationship between intraoperative cultures during hip arthroplasty, obesity, and the risk of early prosthetic joint infection: a prospective study of 428 patients. *Int J Artif Organs*. 2011;34(9):870–5.

Hwang JS, Kim SJ, Bamne AB, Na YG, Kim TK. Do glycaemic markers predict occurrence of complications after total knee arthroplasty in patients with diabetes? *Clin Orthop Relat Res*. 2015;473(5):1726–31.

Jamsen E, Nevalainen P, Eskelinen A, Huotari K, Kalliovaklkama J, Moilanen T. Obesity, diabetes and preoperative hypoglycaemia as predictors of periprosthetic joint infection. A single-centre analysis of 7181 primary hip and knee replacements for osteoarthritis. *J Bone Joint Surg (Am)*. 2012;94:e10:1–9.

Meehan JP, Danielsen B, Kim SH, Jamali AA, White RH. Younger age is associated with a higher risk of early periprosthetic joint infection and aseptic mechanical failure after total knee arthroplasty. *J Bone Joint Surg (Am)*. 2014;96(7):529–35.

Menon TJ, Wroblewski BM. Charnley low-friction arthroplasty in patients with psoriasis. *Clin Orthop Relat Res*. 1983;176:127–8.

Papadopoulos EC, Parvizi J, Lai CH, Lewallen DG. Total knee arthroplasty following prior distal femoral fracture. *Knee*. 2002;9(4):267–74.

Ravi B, Escott B, Shah PS, et al. A systematic review and meta-analysis comparing complications following total joint arthroplasty for rheumatoid arthritis versus for osteoarthritis. *Arthritis Rheum*. 2012;6(12):3839–49.

Rodriguez-Merchan EC. Review article: risk factors of infection following total knee arthroplasty: a systematic review. *J Orthop Surg (Hong Kong)*. 2012;20(2):236–8.

Roffi RP, Merritt PO. Total knee replacement after fractures about the knee. *Orthop Rev*. 1990;19(7):614–20.

Santaguida PL, Hawker GA, Hudak PL, et al. Patient characteristics affecting the prognosis of total hip and knee joint arthroplasty: a systematic review. Review article. *Can J Surg*. 2008;51(6):428–36.

Scharma JC, Espehaug B, Hallan G, et al. Risk of revision for infection in primary total hip and knee arthroplasty in patients with rheumatoid arthritis compared with osteoarthritis: a prospective, population-based study on 108,786 hip and knee joint arthroplasties from the Norwegian Arthroplasty Register. *Arthritis Care Res (Hoboken)*. 2010;62(4):473–9.

Stern SH, Insall JN. Total knee arthroplasty in obese patients. *J Bone Joint Surg (Am)*. 1990;72(9):1400–4.

Suzuki G, Saito S, Ishii T, Motojima S, Tokuhashi Y, Ryu J. Previous fracture surgery is a major risk factor of infection after total knee arthroplasty. *Knee Surg Sports Traumatol Arthrosc*. 2011;19(12):2040–4.

Weiss NG, Parvizi J, Trousdale RT, Bryce RD, Lewallen DG. Total knee arthroplasty in patients with prior fracture of the tibial plateau. *J Bone Joint Surg (Am)*. 2003;85-A(2):218–21.

Chapter 3

Preoperative assessment

The aim of preoperative assessment should be to reduce the risks of prosthetic joint infection (PJI) as well as to enhance postoperative recovery. Risk assessment begins with a detailed history, including previous trauma around the joint to be replaced, diabetic control (as evidenced by the level of HbA1c) and body mass index (BMI). Complications after any previous other joint arthroplasty should alert the clinician to a higher risk of PJI. If it is found that diabetic control has been poor then an effort must be made to correct this. If the patient is a smoker then recruitment to the National Health Service (NHS) quit line *must* be made and if the patient is morbidly obese recruitment onto a weight-loss programme via the general practitioner *must* be made. Both of these independent high-risk variables can be improved preincision.

A specialist PJI team should consist of both *core* and *extended* members.

The core members of the PJI team should ideally be co-located in one hospital and consist of:

1. Specialist orthopaedic surgeon.

2. Specialist plastic surgeon.

3. Microbiologist.

These core members should be supported by specialized nurses and physiotherapists.

Extended members represent specialists who are occasionally called upon for assistance. The extended members of the PJI team are:

1. Vascular surgeon.

2. Limb fitting/rehabilitation centre.

It is acknowledged that some hospitals will already have these teams. For example, major trauma centres (MTCs) should have an Ortho-Plastic team who work closely with microbiologists. Also Vascular networks often have the hub at an MTC. However, if such teams do not exist then it is suggested that networks involving the core and extended members are established. The East Midlands Network has suggested a method of empowering treating surgeons who diagnose a PJI in their patients (see Chapter 8).

Accurate assessment of risk will allow prospective patients to be appropriately counselled about the risk of PJI. A safe pathway is suggested below in the section on 'A safe flow chart in the preoperative assessment for major joint arthroplasty in the lower limb'.

Assessing risk factors for prosthetic joint replacement

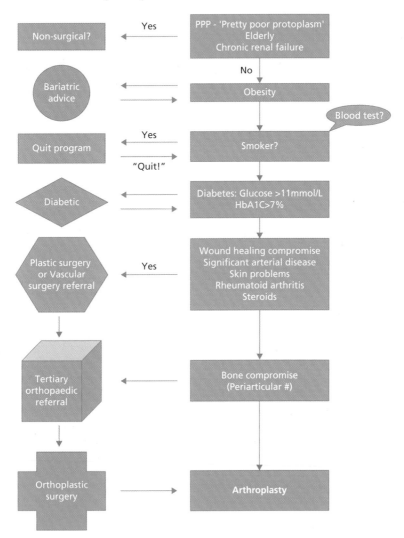

Assessing risk factors for prosthetic
joint replacement

Clinical examination should aim to assess the quality of the skin through which access for the arthropasty is contemplated and a comprehensive clinical assessment of the vascular supply of the limb. Any skin ulceration should be a 'red flag' sign of poor vascularity and provides a source of bacteria with infective potential (see section on Vascular issues for major joint replacement, below).

Vascular issues for major joint replacement

Although some degree of atherosclerosis is ubiquitous in the demographic undergoing elective arthroplasty, the severity of the arterial insufficiency is widely variable and many patients will be asymptomatic since their activity will also be limited by their musculoskeletal disease. Specific risk factors for peripheral arterial disease (PAD) should be assessed in the preoperative history and include, in approximate ranking of importance:

- Smoking
- Diabetes
- Family history of PAD, ischaemic heart disease or stroke
- Male gender
- Increasing age
- Hypertension
- Hypercholesterolaemia.

Although some of these factors are modifiable, in the timeframe for arthroplasty the main benefit of addressing these is related to anaesthetic fitness. Longer term benefits in life expectancy are related to slowing the progression of the PAD and avoiding the cardiac and cerebrovascular complications. Significant improvement in peripheral arterial circulation usually requires radiological or surgical intervention.

PAD in the UK is predominantly atherosclerotic in origin and occlusive in nature, but clinicians should be alert to rarer forms of vascular disease, including popliteal aneurysms, connective tissue disorders, or vascular malformations affecting the operative site.

Atherosclerosis is a universal, systemic, slowly progressive degenerative condition of the wall of major arteries, which gradually narrows the lumen and restricts bloodflow. This process is balanced by the gradual development of collaterals and the reduced need for muscular activity with age, such that many patients remain asymptomatic even in the presence of demonstrable disease. Increasing age, male gender, genetic factors (family history), smoking, diabetes, hypertension, and hyperlipidaemia are factors associated with the development of more severe disease.

The majority of PAD affects the lower limbs, as with degenerative joint disease, and it is very common in the population who are likely to be considered for arthroplasty—up to 15% of men over 65 years will have clinically detectable PAD (Fitridge and Thompson, 2007), as demonstrated by absent pedal pulses. A smaller proportion will have symptoms of aching calf muscles on walking that resolve swiftly on resting (intermittent claudication), and a few will progress to critical limb ischaemia (CLI), as evidenced by non-healing ulcers, necrotic toes, or rest pain in the foot.

Patients with CLI should be seen and assessed by a vascular surgeon prior to arthroplasty. It is likely that revascularization will be appropriate to save the limb and this may preclude the joint operation.

In the absence of CLI, most patients with PAD will have developed a collateral circulation owing to the slow progression of the arterial disease, and this will be adequate both for their day-to-day needs and for wound healing.

An absent femoral pulse is a significant finding and will raise the risk of pressure area ulceration and poor wound healing. Patients with an absent femoral pulse should be referred to a vascular surgeon preoperatively for investigation and intervention.

It will be rare that infrainguinal revascularization will be appropriate before lower limb arthroplasty if a femoral pulse is present.

Risk assessment for vascular complications

Risk assessment for vascular complications should include:

- Comorbidities, including diabetes, prominent bony abnormality in pressure area, smoking, neuropathy, ischaemic heart disease.
- Previous vascular interventions on ipsilateral and contralateral limb.
- Palpable pulses: document presence or absence of femoral and pedal (posterior tibial [PT], dorsalis pedis [DP]) pulses. A single palpable foot pulse is sufficient.
  - Assessment of the popliteal pulse is difficult, especially with soft-tissue changes around the knee. If a popliteal pulse can be easily felt, consider a duplex scan to exclude a popliteal aneurysm.
- If no foot pulses are palpable, then a hand-held Doppler (HHD) assessment is useful, but palpation of the femoral pulse is mandatory.
- Ankle:brachial pressure index (ABPI) if no foot pulses palpable. Although unlikely to indicate vascular intervention, patients are at high risk for pressure area breakdown if ABPI <0.5.

The presence of leg ulceration merits formal vascular laboratory arterial and venous assessments before arthroplasty.

A safe flow chart in the preoperative assessment for major joint arthroplasty in the lower limb

Safety flow chart for pre-operative assessment

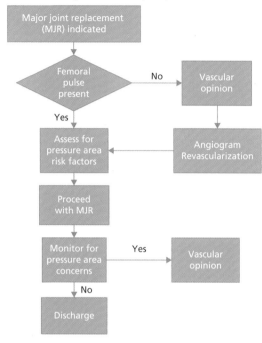

If there is no femoral pulse preoperatively, a vascular opinion *must* be sought before lower limb arthroplasty surgery as iliac disease can usually be treated by angioplasty/stenting and will reduce the risks of both wound healing and pressure area problems.

If angioplasty is undertaken, patients can safely undergo arthroplasty after 6 months (often patients may be on anti-platelet therapy, which will need to be stopped).

The potential vascular problems during and after major joint replacement (MJR) fall into several categories:

- Acute limb ischaemia
- Vascular injury
- General cardiovascular considerations
- Pressure area ulceration.

Acute limb ischaemia

Acute critical ischaemia postoperatively is rare in the absence of vascular trauma and occurs in less than 0.5% of total knee replacements (Abu Dakka et al., 2009). Potential causes of acute limb ischaemia include vessel injury, thrombosis in situ, occlusion of a previous bypass graft, or thrombosis/embolism related to a popliteal aneurysm. However, the classic symptoms (Box 3.1) may be absent in postoperative patients and a high index of suspicion based on signs is advised.

The window of opportunity to rescue muscle from ischaemic necrosis is only a few hours. Bloodflow can be restored beyond this timepoint; however, irreparable tissue damage will have already occurred and the limb cannot be saved. Also, reperfusion may be fatal beyond this point owing to the release of toxins, including myoglobin, into the circulation. A metabolic acidosis ensues, causing acute renal failure, cardiac arrhythmias, and adult respiratory distress syndrome. Calling for an opinion from a vascular surgeon as early as possible may mean the difference between a vascular salvage and an amputation.

Epidural anaesthesia effectively masks the motor and sensory symptoms of vascular insufficiency; higher importance is therefore placed on the appearance of the limbs and pulse status. Similarly, analgesia and the lack of mobility and pain from the operation site may obscure symptoms.

An HHD should be available in every postoperative recovery area, and all surgeons performing MJR should be competent to use HHD to identify foot pulses

Ischaemia owing to vessel injury may be related to arterial ligation, division with spasm (there may be surprisingly little bleeding), traction, or intimal dissection. It

---

Box 3.1 Classic symptoms of acute limb ischaemia

Pain
Paraesthesia
Paralysis
Pallor
Perishing cold
Pulselessness

may be apparent only at the end of the procedure from the appearance of the limb. Compare the appearance and examination of the limb with the preoperative status and, if needed, call for vascular input before the patient leaves theatre. The absence of foot pulses that were clearly documented preoperatively is an important indication of major arterial compromise.

In-situ thrombosis of native arteries is remarkably uncommon despite the high prevalence of coexistent arterial and joint disease. The collateral circulation that these patients have developed over the years is generally resistant to both position and tourniquet use and is adequate to keep the limb viable.

The presence of a previous bypass graft should be evident from the history and specifically sought. The presence of scars over the groin and medial thigh/calf should alert the clinician to the possibility of an underlying graft. Occlusion of a bypass graft is more likely if the limb is flexed at the hip or knee for prolonged periods, or a tourniquet is used such that a previous infrainguinal bypass graft in the limb for MJR is a contraindication for use of a tourniquet. A prosthetic graft is much more likely to occlude than a vein graft, and a bypass crossing the knee joint is less resilient than one to the above-knee artery. If in doubt, ask for a vascular opinion.

Popliteal aneurysms are rare, but should be considered if the popliteal pulse is readily palpable, especially if asymmetrically so. There is an association with abdominal aortic aneurysm (AAA), and the history of a previous AAA repair should raise a red flag. Duplex ultrasound is the definitive test. Popliteal aneurysms are prone to thrombosis owing to flexion of the knee or a tourniquet, and will produce severe acute ischaemia very rapidly as no collateral circulation has been developed.

Vascular injury

Vascular injury may be arterial or venous—both can be life-threatening. Arterial injury may lead to bleeding or ischaemia (see section on Acute limb ischaemia above).

Bleeding may be occult or overt, arterial or venous, intraoperative or postoperative. The immediate management of unexpected intraoperative bleeding should be local pressure with a swab and call for vascular surgeon input. Try to resist the temptation to put big clamps on blindly.

Significant postoperative bleeding will be manifest by a large amount of drainage or a progressive swelling. Development of a haematoma in a confined space may lead to ischaemia of the more distal portion of the limb. Unless the patient is haemodynamically unstable, a call for vascular input before reopening the wound would be prudent as simple release of the incision site will release the tamponade effect and may result in profuse haemorrhage. On occasion the swelling will become evident after the procedure during the following few days, in which case there is opportunity for investigation with duplex, computed tomography and/or angiography, which may allow radiological intervention to control the bleeding point.

General cardiovascular considerations

Anti-platelet therapy should be discontinued as late as possible and restarted as soon as possible, particularly if a prosthetic bypass graft is present. Patients with clinically apparent PAD have a 30% risk of a myocardial or cerebrovascular event within 5 years after arterial reconstruction and these are more common after any subsequent surgery.

Pressure area ulceration

Pressure area ulceration, like deep vein thrombosis, often begins during the operation, and is exacerbated by postoperative immobility. Almost all ulceration is preventable in an elective patient of independent mobility preoperatively. The bony prominences of the heel, sacrum, and greater trochanter are prone to locally impaired skin circulation in immobile patients with cachexia or obesity.

Even a normal circulation may not protect against development of pressure area problems, but both the risk of development and the likelihood and speed of healing are directly related to the degree of coexistent arterial disease. Simple pressure-relieving measures (mattresses, boots, etc.) should be used and vascular input requested if the condition is not improving. Vascular intervention may be required to expedite healing.

Skin compromise in proximal (greater trochanter and sacrum) areas is primarily related to local pressure issues if a femoral pulse is palpable.

PAD will predominantly increase the risk of the more distal pressure areas. The dorsum of the foot and the medial and lateral metatarsal heads may develop significant impairment of local perfusion in the presence of bandaging and subsequent lower limb swelling. This will be exacerbated by PAD.

There are well-documented risk factors, including PAD (Waterlow, 2005), which increase the incidence of pressure-related problems and should be assessed routinely preoperatively. All hospitals should have a protocol for graduated care of patients at increased risk.

Amputation and rehabilitation

Despite the best efforts of the multidisciplinary team, there will be occasions when the PJI cannot be controlled and the patient has significant symptoms, leading to a poor quality of life. On a case-by-case basis such patients should be assessed for major amputation with prosthetic limb replacement where possible.

The National Confidential Enquiry into Patient Outcome and Death (NCEPOD) report (2014) on amputation services makes the following recommendations relevant to PJI:

A multidisciplinary team should care for all major amputation patients and should include: surgeons, physiotherapists, occupational therapists, specialist nurses, and rehabilitation specialists under the care of a single named clinician (Vascular

Society of Great Britain and Ireland, 2016). This team should be supported by diabetologists, clinical psychologists, anaesthetists, microbiologists, acute pain service, and other relevant specialist teams.

Selection of the level of amputation is part of the multidisciplinary team process.

Consultant level input is central to optimal results, and procedures should be carried out on elective consultant lists.

Discharge planning should commence when the need for amputation is identified and is led by a complex discharge coordinator.

These services are best developed in centres with vascular surgery on site, since chronic ischaemia is the single commonest cause of limb loss in the UK adult population at present. There is a clear volume:outcome relationship with amputation (as with most operations) in terms of optimal limb length preservation and healing. Consideration should be given to referring such patients to the vascular team, because of the established links and greater experience with major amputation, as this is associated with better outcomes overall in terms of stump healing. At centres performing a large number of revision joints where there is sufficient demand from the PJI programme, there may be value in one of the PJI multidisciplinary surgical teams taking the lead for these cases, using the same pathways as for vascular amputees.

References

Abu Dakka M, Badri H, Al-Khaffaf H. Total knee arthroplasty in patients with peripheral vascular disease. *Surgeon*. 2009;7(6):362–5.

Fitridge R, Thompson M. *Mechanisms of Vascular Disease: A Textbook for Vascular Surgeons.* Cambridge: Cambridge University Press, 2007.

National Confidential Enquiry into Patient Outcome and Death. *Lower Limb Amputation: Working Together,* 2014. http://www.ncepod.org.uk/2014lla.html

Vascular Society of Great Britain and Ireland. *Quality Improvement Framework for Major Amputation Surgery,* April 2016. https://www.vascularsociety.org.uk/_userfiles/pages/files/Resources/Vasc_Soc_Amputation_Paper_V2.pdf

Waterlow J. *The Waterlow Pressure Ulcer Prevention Manual.*(Revised 2005). http://www.judy-waterlow.co.uk/the-waterlow-manual.htm

Chapter 4

Thromboprophylaxis and haematomas

Venous thromboprophylaxis remains a topical and contentious issue for arthroplasty surgeons. Whereas it is accepted that there is a real need to minimize deep venous thrombosis (DVT) and pulmonary embolism (PE), haematoma formation and persistent wound leakage as a consequence of thromboprophylaxis carry their own substantial risks for patients.

An estimated 25,000 people in the UK die from preventable hospital-acquired venous thromboembolism (VTE) every year (House of Commons Health Committee, 2005). Reducing the risk of VTE (DVT and PE) in patients admitted to hospital has been a clinical and political priority. Additionally, the treatment of non-fatal symptomatic VTE and related long-term morbidities is associated with considerable cost to the health service. Guidelines published by The National Institute for Clinical Excellence in January 2010 have led the debate in the UK. VTE risk factors are well known and are listed in Box 4.1.

Assessing risk of VTE before surgery is therefore mandatory, and both surgical and trauma patients should be regarded as being at increased risk if:

- Total anaesthetic and surgical time is >90 min.
- Total anaesthetic and surgical time is 60 min if surgery involves the pelvis or lower limb.
- Acute admission—inflammatory condition.
- Expected significant reduction in mobility.
- One or more of the risk factors in Box 4.1 is present.

Significantly reduced mobility is defined as bedbound, unable to walk unaided, or likely to spend a substantial proportion of the day in bed or in a chair.

Reducing the risk of VTE includes preventing dehydration and encouraging mobilization as soon as clinically safe and possible. Pharmacological and mechanical VTE prophylaxis should be offered to patients at risk, and should continue until the patient is no longer at increased risk of VTE. Mechanical VTE prophylaxis should be chosen based on the clinical condition, surgical procedure, and patient preference. The options include anti-embolism stockings (thigh or knee length), foot impulse devices, and intermittent pneumatic compression devices. The choice of pharmacological VTE prophylaxis should be based on local policies, clinical condition (for example, renal failure), and patient preference, and should be decided locally at a multidisciplinary level involving surgeon, pharmacist, and haematologist.

Significant morbidity is associated with large haematomas and persistent wound leakage, both of which can complicate pharmacological thromboprophylaxis. All

Box 4.1 Venous thromboembolism risk factors

Cancer or cancer treatment
Age >60 years
Critical care admission
Dehydration
Known thrombophilias
Body mass index >30
Venous thromboembolism history
Use of hormone replacement therapy
Use of oestrogen oral contraceptive pills
Varicosed veins with phlebitis
Lower limb surgery
Prolonged immobility
Smoking

patients should be assessed for an increased risk of bleeding before offering pharmacological VTE prophylaxis. Unless the risk of VTE outweighs the risk of bleeding, pharmacological thromboprophylaxis should be withheld in high-risk patients. Equally, in the postoperative period, significant and continued wound leakage or haematoma should indicate the need to stop pharmacological thromboprophylaxis. Prolonged wound drainage after primary total hip arthroplasty is associated with low molecular-weight heparin use and results in increased infection rates (Patel et al., 2007), and anticoagulation with warfarin has a higher risk of deep joint infection (9% versus 2.2%), haematoma/wound ooze (28% versus 4%), and superficial infection (13.5% versus 2.2%), compared with other modalities of thromboprophylaxis (McDougall et al., 2013). Evacuation of a postoperative haematoma after primary total knee arthroplasty within 30 days of index surgery leads to significant sequelae. In patients with this complication, Galat et al. (2008) reported a 2-year cumulative probability of undergoing subsequent major surgery (component resection, muscle flap, or amputation) of 12.3% and of developing a deep infection of 10.5%.

Conclusions

It is suggested that, when assessing patients for arthroplasty, all risk factors are taken into account prior to surgery. It is also suggested that, when there are a number of risk factors in the same patient, referral to a clinic with both core and extended members may help in preventing a prosthetic joint infection.

References

Galat DD, McGovern SC, Hanssen AD, Larson DR, Harrington JR, Clarke HD. Early return to surgery for evacuation of a postoperative haematoma after primary total knee arthroplasty. *J Bone Joint Surg Am.* 2008;90(11):2331–6.

House of Commons Health Committee. *The Prevention of Venous Thromboembolism in Hospitalised Patients*, 2005. London: The Stationery Office Ltd.

McDougall CJ, Gray HS, Simpson PM, Whitehouse SL, Crawford RW, Donnelly WJ. Complications related to therapeutic anticoagulation in total hip arthroplasty. *J Arthroplasty*. 2013;28(1):187–92.

Patel VP, Walsh M, Sehegal B, Preston C, DeWal H, Di Cesare PE. Factors associated with prolonged wound drainage after primary total hip and knee arthroplasty. *J Bone Joint Surg Am*. 2007;89(1):33–8.

The National Institute for Health and Care Excellence. *Venous Thromboembolism: Reducing the Risk*. January 2010. London: NICE.

Chapter 5

Considering safe patient pathways

This group examined three specific clinical senarios for which safe pathways were considered. These are:

1. Necrotic skin—post-arthoplasty.
2. Established prosthetic joint infection (PJI).
3. A combination of points 1 and 2.

Skin necrosis

The skin incision may dehisce despite a non-infected arthroplasty. This is often due to ischaemia, which itself is a result of poor tissue handling during the procedure. There are basic principles that reduce this risk. Safe access to the underlying joint via the integument is outlined.

Safe raising of fasciocutaneous flaps around the joints

The joints of human limbs are surrounded by a variable thickness of soft tissue (integument, muscle, and tendon). Those that are surrounded by muscle groups (shoulder and hip) are relatively well protected when compared with the elbow, wrist, knee, and ankle. Safe access to these more vulnerable joints may be difficult. Difficulties arise when there has been previous surgery (elective or emergency) or when primary surgery is being undertaken on a severely deformed joint. The knee is the largest synovial joint in the body and is comparatively superficial. The integument is thin and pliable. The distal femoral metaphysis and the proximal tibial metaphysis contain the growth plates in an immature skeleton. As a result of this, the skin surrounding the knee benefits by receiving a blood supply that is constant and reliable. Most of the feeding vessels travel just deep to or are within the deep fascia. The fascia around superficial joints such as the knee and elbow is well developed and separates the integument from the gliding surfaces, where relative motion occurs during flexion/extension. Safe planning and execution is thus afforded when the skin flaps are thick with little undermining. Should undermining be necessary, then care must be taken to ensure that the skin edges are never crushed and that any lateral dissection respects the perforating vessels, which pierce the fascia from the main feeder vessels to nourish the skin flaps.

Tips and tricks to avoid iatrogenic skin necrosis

Avoid extensive undermining

This should be intuitive since these flaps of skin are fed by random feeder vessels within the substance of the base of the flaps, which perforate into the subcutaneous tissue and then skin. Inadvertent sacrifice of these vessels will diminish the circulation. This will have a negative additive effect on the patient's ability to heal at the incision site. It is, however, conceded that the patient demographic for arthoplasty may render the accurate identification of tissue planes difficult; nonetheless, restricting the extent of undermining of the access skin flaps to allow (for example) medial/lateral release of soft tissues in varus/valgus joints should prevent ischaemia of the incision site. The ischaemia is independent of tension of closure of the skin.

Avoid sharp changes in the direction of the skin incision(s)

Acute changes in the direction of an incision can potentially leave ischaemic tips of the skin incision and are usually considered when one is dealing with arthroplasty after previous open joint surgery or after open trauma around the joint.

Avoid ending up with long, thin apical skin segments

The principles for avoiding apical segments of skin flaps are the same as for avoiding acute changes in the direction of skin incision. If sharp, long, pointy tips are present then elective excision of these is recommended to avoid scabs of dry necrosis appearing several days/weeks after arthroplasty.

Sham incisions can be of some value. These work by preconditioning the skin flaps to the intended line(s) of election for arthroplasty (Jonsson et al., 1988; Barthe Garcia et al., 1991). Sham incisions should be made a minimum of 3 weeks prior to definitive surgery. It should be noted that, although these will be indicative of wound healing problems, a well-healed sham incision cannot guarantee problem-free healing. This is because a true 'delay phenomenon' requires more extensive dissection of the skin flap than a surgical incision.

Elbow

The elbow joint is similar (in terms of soft tissue surrounding it) to the knee joint but is rotated 180° in its axis. It thus has the major neurovascular structures on the anterior aspect and a pliable, thin bursa and skin on the posterior surface. The distal humerus and the proximal ulna grow less than the respective opposite ends. This is reflected in the relative paucity of dependable cutaneous blood vessels. A collateral blood circulation exists around the elbow joint. Collateral, recurrent vessels form circulating anastomotic connections between the radial and ulnar arteries. These vessels give off perforating arteries through the fascia into the skin along the lateral and medial axes of the humeral epicondyles. Thus midline posterior incisions are safe as long as the deep fascia is raised with the skin flaps should undermining be required. These incisions become precarious when there has been previous surgery to the medial or lateral aspect of the elbow joint or any previous trauma.

Ankle

The ankle joint is a sophisticated hinge-type joint, which allows the articulation of the plafond of the tibia on the dome of the talus. The lateral malleolus affords some intrinsic stability. There are soft-tissue structures, which add extrinsic stability. Like the elbow joint, however, the skin surrounding the joint derives its blood supply from axial named vessels. There are few predictable perforating vessels. The concept of 'angiosomes' (Taylor and Palmer, 1987; Morris and Taylor, 1993) needs to be studied to understand the territories of the skin around the ankle, which are separately supplied by differing, named vessels.

Prosthetic joint infection negative-pressure dressings to reduce risk

Some investigators have suggested that applying a negative-pressure dressing over a surgical incision improves incision healing. These studies were undertaken in high-risk post-trauma incisions (Stannard et al., 2012). Others have investigated the evidence for negative pressure dressing in reducing the rate of surgical site infection (SSI; Walter et al., 2012). The conclusion was that there was no influence on SSI by negative-pressure dressing. Negative-pressure dressing may reduce the seroma rate after total hip replacement (Pachowsky et al., 2012). Elective negative-pressure dressing was not recommended following arthroplasty.

This group believes that the use of negative-pressure dressing after arthroplasty is not indicated based on the current literature.

If skin necrosis occur despite care and attention to the technique detailed above, then a safe pathway must be sought for effective management.

Pathway for skin necrosis

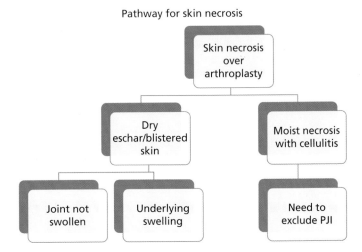

Pathway for skin necrosis

If the skin necrosis is dry without cellulitis and there is no underlying joint swelling, then it is likely that the necrosis is due to ischaemia of the skin flaps and, as such, will be expected to be extracapsular. Such patients can be managed by plastic surgeons with simple techniques in the majority of cases.

The other two scenarios must raise suspicions of PJI and this must be excluded. This can be done locally. The modality by which this is done is determined by the treating orthopaedic surgeon. With a swollen joint an aspiration is indicated, whether done with the assistance of ultrasound or not. It is suggested that this aspiration is performed in theatre conditions. Testing of joint aspirate for white blood cells as well as chemical analysis should then be undertaken.

If the tests are equivocal then excision of the necrotic skin is undertaken together with evacuation of any haematoma. Haematomas are not uncommon after arthroplasty and cause skin necrosis by a number of mechanisms. The physical impingement of the skin flaps by an expanding haematoma will cause ischaemia directly. Indirectly, unrelieved haematomas cause cellular toxicity by generation of free radicals (Glass and Nanchahal, 2012).

If the necrosis is extracapsular then the necrotic skin is excised. A negative-pressure dressing can then be applied to temporize the wound until reconstruction.

The pathway below illustrates the typical scenarios following examination under anaesthetic (EUA).

Pathway for scenarios following examination under anaesthetic

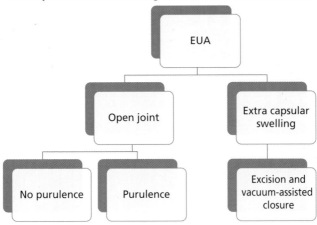

If no purulence is detected with the naked eye and sterility confirmed by microbiology then PJI has been excluded. Some advocate a liner exchange for such arthroplasty devices that allow this (see Chapter 6). When there is frank purulence then referral to an Ortho-Plastic centre is recommended.

References

Barthe Garcia P, Suarez Nieto C, Rojo Ortega JM. Morphological changes in the vascularisation of delayed flaps in rabbits. *Br J Plast Surg.* 1991;44(4):285–90.

Glass GE, Nanchahal J. Why haematomas cause flap failure: an evidence-based paradigm. *J Plast Reconstr Aesthet Surg.* 2012;65(7):903–10.

Jonsson K, Hunt TK, Brennan SS, Mathes SJ. Tissue oxygen measurements in delayed skin flaps: a reconsideration of the mechanisms of the delay phenomenon. *Plast Reconstr Surg.* 1988;82(2):328–36.

Morris SF, Taylor GI. Predicting the survival of experimental skin flaps with a knowledge of the vascular architecture. *Plast Reconstr Surg.* 1993;92(7):1352–61.

Pachowsky M, Gusinde J, Klein A, et al. Negative pressure wound therapy to prevent seromas and treat surgical incisions after total hip arthroplasty. *Orthop.* 2012;36(4):719–22.

Stannard JP, Volgas DA, McGwin G, et al. Incisional negative pressure wound therapy after high-risk lower extremity fractures. *J Orthop Trauma.* 2012;26(1):37–42.

Taylor GI, Palmer JH. The vascular territories (angiosomes) of the body: experimental study and clinical application. *Br J Plast Surg.* 1987;40(2):113–41.

Walter CJ, Dumville JC, Sharp CA, Page T. Systematic review and meta-analysis of wound dressings in the prevention of surgical-site infections (SSI) in surgical wounds healing by primary intention. *Br J Surg.* 2012;99(9):1185–94.

Chapter 6

Pathways for established prosthetic joint infection

When there is an obvious prosthetic joint infection (PJI) (see Chapter 1) then referral to a core of specialists is recommended. The management of infected arthroplasty is variable, with different approaches reported in the literature. It is also important to differentiate between the management of an acutely infected implant and that of low-grade infection. This section will therefore address both of these conditions separately.

Management of acute infection

Diagnosis

The diagnosis of an acute infection following total joint replacement surgery is usually obvious (see Chapter 1). The patient will usually present with systemic upset, fever, and pain in the replaced joint, and obvious signs of local infection. This will be accompanied by tachycardia, potential changes in blood pressure and raised temperature. Haematological investigations will usually show a significantly raised C-reactive protein, a raised white count with other haematological changes possibly, depending on the severity of the infection.

Initial management

Initial management of these patients should focus on resuscitation and general principles of management of acute sepsis. All patients should have an intravenous infusion, be placed on regular observations to monitor pulse, blood pressure, temperature, and urine output, and the infected joint should be aspirated without delay to allow microbiological evaluation of the underlying bacteria. Once aspiration has been performed, empiric antibiotics should be commenced (microbiologist to advise).

Surgical management of acute infection

Arthroscopic debridement

Arthroscopic surgery, particularly for acute knee infections following total knee replacement, can be useful in the management of acutely ill patients to decrease the septic load and to allow early resuscitation and prompt diagnosis. Arthroscopic surgery, however, has no role in the definitive treatment of an acutely infected joint replacement. If arthroscopy is used for the above reasons it must be followed by open definitive surgery.

Implant retention strategies

If the infection is acute (either within the first few weeks of joint replacement surgery or the patient presents with an acute haematogenous infection some time after surgery but has well-fixed implants), then implant retention can be achieved in as many as 70–80% of cases—the so-called debridement, antibiotics, and implant retention (DAIR) procedure (Byren et al., 2009). The principles of this treatment depend on having specialist microbiology advice coupled with early aggressive surgical intervention.

The surgical procedure must include an open arthrotomy, extensive debridement of all infected material, and a full synovectomy. All modular components within the articulation should be removed and the interface cleaned thoroughly prior to reimplantation. The whole area needs to be fully debrided and irrigated with copious amounts of clean fluid. Multiple samples taken using the 'no-touch' technique should always be sent to the laboratory to confirm the underlying organism and antimicrobial sensitivities.

Postoperatively high-dose intravenous antibiotics are given as prescribed by the microbiologist for the network. A PICC (peripherally inserted central catheter) line is usually required to allow antibiotics to be given in high enough dose, initially at least, and these can be given in an outpatient setting provided that an OPAT (outpatient antibiotic therapy) service is available. Intravenous antibiotics may be followed by oral antibiotics. The duration of such treatment is currently the subject of considerable debate, with some centres advocating a minimum of 6 months.

Formal revision surgery

Formal revision surgery—either one-stage or two-stage—can also be performed in the acute setting or following failure of a DAIR procedure. The same principles as described above apply but will include removal of all the implants and reimplantation either as a one-stage or two-stage procedure. Much debate remains regarding what defines a one-stage procedure, the interval between first and second stage, spacer use between stages and the duration of antibiotic therapy following each stage. These are matters for the local regional networks to discuss.

Management of chronic low-grade infection

A significant number of infected arthroplasties present late with chronic low-grade infection. These are usually as a result of infection such as coagulase-negative staphylococcus, but other bacteria can be implicated. The treatment principles depend on early diagnosis and will also vary depending on the underlying infective organism. Perhaps paradoxically, the biology of such chronic infections, always involving considerable bacterial biofilm formation, makes for a considerable failure rate, as such organisms will be intrinsically resistant to all antibiotics targeting the cell wall as well as several other classes of anti-infective agent. Microbiology input is mandatory for such cases.

Diagnosis

The diagnosis of a chronic low-grade infection can be difficult. A useful document to aid in this is the *Proceedings of the International Consensus meeting on Periprosthetic Joint Infection* (Gehrke and Parvizi, 2013). Chapter 7 covers the most up-to-date review of published literature on the diagnosis of PJI infection.

Role of aspiration

Aspiration is an important consideration in all total joint replacements where infection is suspected. Whilst not 100% accurate, aspiration does allow identification of the infecting organism in as many as 75% of cases (Gehrke and Parvizi, 2013). New diagnostic technologies such as Synovasure™ are also now available and depend on the presence of alpha-defensin within the aspirate. This appears to have good positive predictive test performance for infection but does nothing to identify the relevant organism and its antimicrobial sensitivy pattern. Their role is currently unclear but initial results appear promising.

Management of low-grade infection

Of primary importance in this situation is assessment of the underlying soft-tissue envelope as this is often compromised in patients with severe chronic low-grade infection. The presence of sinuses and other soft-tissue problems should prompt early plastic surgical opinion before reconstructive surgery is contemplated.

Once a plan for the soft-tissue envelope is made, formal revision surgery is the only method of eradication of infection. This can be performed on a one- or two-stage basis. All infected arthroplasties should be managed within a specialist centre where specialized microbiology advice, plastic surgical input, and specific orthopaedic expertise are available. The choice between one-stage or two-stage revision surgery will depend on a number of factors and will include the relevant expertise available in the treating centre, the availability of a specialist microbiology service, and the nature of the underlying organism.

Antibiotic suppression

Antibiotic suppression should not be a treatment of choice for infected joint replacement. The mainstay of treatment has to be surgical to eradicate the infection. In a small number of cases, however, and in particular if the patient is not able to survive major surgical intervention, suppression of the infection with long-term antibiotics can be considered but only as a last resort. Similarly, patients unfit for surgery may be managed without major surgical intervention by allowing a sinus to drain freely and using intermittent antibiotic courses as clinically indicated (sinus persistence).

Flap algorithm for patients with prosthetic joint infection

Flap Algorithm for PJI patients

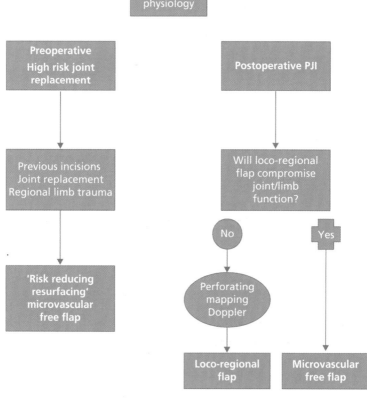

Soft-tissue reconstruction

1. Around the shoulder.

   When PJI complicates shoulder arthroplasty undertaken via an anterior incision, the implant can be removed; enough skin laxity exists with a robust vascularity that primary closure is comparatively easy to achieve. In those cases where there are multiple sinuses and/or there has been previous surgery due to trauma, then flap cover is indicated. Local flaps are reliable around the shoulder (Davami and Porkhamene, 2011). The tissue from the back based on the subscapular vascular axis can be harvested and delivered into an anterior defect. Both fasciocutaneous flaps (scapular and parascapular) as well as muscle flaps (latissimus dorsi and serratus anterior) may be used. The fasciocutaneous flaps carry less morbidity and are recommended.

2. Around the elbow.

   An important consideration for local tissue transfer is the identification and protection of the ulnar nerve. Local flaps are less reliable and one often resorts to pedicled fasciocutaneous flaps. A traditional flap is the radial forearm flap based on the radial artery and its comitant veins. Similarly, the ulnar artery can be used as the source vessel for tissue transfer from the ulnar border of the forearm. Tissue from the lateral arm, based upon the posterior radial recurrent artery and its comitant veins, can be used occasionally as there is said to be less of a donor site issue when compared with the radial and ulnar forearm flaps (Adkinson and Chung, 2014). Care must be taken when tunnelling the flap pedicle into the defect to avoid injury to the main nerves around the elbow.

3. Around the wrist.

   Wrist arthroplasty is not common as fusion is often favoured. However, when required even for wound closure after fusion the use of local flaps is recommended. Again, the use of the radial forearm tissue based on the radial artery and its comitant veins can be relied upon but in a reverse fashion. The prerequisite for this flap to work is an intact palmar arch. A newer and less morbid flap is the Becker flap, which relies upon a feeding vessel arising from the ulnar artery (Karki and Singh, 2007). Free tissue transfer can be effective as the recipient vessels are reliable and easily found around the wrist.

4. Around the hip.

   Like the shoulder, the hip is surrounded by lax tissue and, often, when undertaking excisional and revisional surgery, the skin can be mobilized upon a robust blood supply and sutured without risk of necrosis. There are, however, occasions when this becomes difficult in, for example, repeated washouts with multiple sinus tracts and in multiple revision cases. Often the reason for multiple operations is a lack of experience by the operating surgeon to excise membrane and undertake a composite tissue excision. After such radical surgery the local tissue is difficult to mobilize predictably and one must resort to importing vascularized tissue. Again, local tissue is preferred and the skin and muscles of the thigh can be effectively used (Choa et al., 2011). Tensor fascia lata flap is less morbid than the rectus and the vastus lateralis, and has the advantage that it can be split. Thus the muscle and fascia are dissected free from the skin and rotated into the defect and anchored to the pelvis. The skin is then sutured tension-free.

5. Around the knee.

Wounds around the knee joint are difficult to reconstruct effectively. This is even more so in the presence of an implant. Some have developed algorithms to help surgeons to decide how best to approach defects around the knee (Laing et al., 1992; Panni et al., 2010). When all high-risk factors have been controlled and a decision made relating to implant retention or otherwise, then consideration should be given to how the soft-tissue defect is to be reconstructed. To help with this important decision the technique used must allow for an easy access for a definitive implant. Thus a skin-grafted area will be less easy than a flap with fasciocutaneous paddle to re-raise safely. Prior to reconstruction the vascular status of the limb must be ascertained.

The following schema should be seen as a guide.

1. A defect over the ligamentum patellae or near its insertion. This is one of the most common defects encountered as a wound complicating total knee replacement. It is also amenable to a pedicled medial gastrocnemius flap. The commonest procedure is to transpose the flap as a muscle-only flap, necessitating a split-thickness skin graft. Accurate planning that takes into account the arc of rotation and insetting must be integral to flap dissection. This will allow a tension-free suturing of the distal part of the flap (the Achilles region of the flap) along the superior aspect of the defect. A small skin paddle can be incorporated with the muscle as a myocutaneous flap. Transmuscular perforators can be seen during harvest to allow a more reliable skin flap. This concept can allow a perforator-based skin-only flap such as the medial sural artery perforator flap (MSAP). Although attractive in the fact that muscle is not harvested, it must be remembered that in cases of knee PJI the capsule of the joint is destroyed either by infection or by excision. As such, the medial head of gastrocnemius fans out under the surrounding skin flaps during insetting. This 'water-proofing' effect may be lost with MSAP flaps. More studies are needed to address the clinical effectiveness of perforator flaps for this defect.

2. Pre-patellar defect. The medial head of gastrocnemius will not reach this area without dis-inserting the origin from the femoral condyle. The latter procedure may need to be coupled with a transverse scoring of the deep aspect of the muscle. Both of these procedures risk devascularizing the flap and thus must be done with due care. A pre-patellar wound can be skin grafted if there is no PJI of the implant underneath and if the periosteum of the patella remains viable. This will allow healing but it must be anticipated that further soft-tissue reconstruction will need to be undertaken. A local fasciocutaneous flap may be planned as a random pattern flap or an MSAP—if the proportions of the calf allow this.

3. Suprapatellar defects. In the presence of a PJI these defects are exceptionally difficult to cover with vascularized tissue. Whereas the vastus muscles may seem

attractive owing to their proximity, the morbidity from their harvest must be taken into account. The distally based gracilis flap may seem counterintuitive since this is a type 2 flap, which theoretically means that it will necrose when the proximal (dominant) pedicle has been ligated, but the distally based gracilis flap has been shown to be reliable, especially when delayed (Tiengo et al., 2011; Mitsala et al., 2014). The pedicled, distally based anterolateral thigh flap has been used by some, but the issue of venous congestion would make this a risky reconstruction (Demirseren et al., 2011).

4. Proximal incisional wound. A redeeming feature here is that this incision is over the quadriceps muscle group plus there is often laxity of the skin, and if primary closure can be undertaken a 'Z'-plasty may help to move the incision away from the defect in the knee extensors.

5. Posterior defects. These are rare. These may occur when there has been previous trauma leading to a weakness in the posterior capsule. Nonetheless, small defects in the popliteal fossa can be excised and closed, primarily with a 'Z'-plasty. For larger defects, random pattern fasciocutaneous flaps can be planned with a proximal 'back-cut'.

Free flaps

Most of the reconstructive options rely on local tissue. This is both quick and effective when planned and executed well. There are, however, defects that are either located in hostile locations (lateral part of the knee joint) or that are too large for local flaps. In these cases free-tissue transfer must be planned. Safe planning relies upon a good donor flap as well as reliable recipient vessels. The large popliteal vessels or proximally the superficial femoral vessels seem obvious choices, but these will need vein grafts to allow realistic pedicle lengths (Cetrulo et al., 2008). The genicular vessels (medial and lateral) are consistent and are of a good calibre (Rees-Lee and Khan, 2011; Wiedner et al., 2011). The great saphenous vein must be used as the venous recipient. Free flaps also allow reconstruction of composite defects (e.g. the knee extensors can be reconstructed at the same time by composite tissue transfer). Free-flap reconstruction must be carefully considered and a preoperative discussion with patients, their relatives, the surgeons, and the anaesthetists must take place to ensure that all are aware of the risks of donor site morbidity and of putting the patient through prolonged surgery and a period of a hyperdynamic circulation.

6. Around the ankle.

Total ankle arthroplasty has gained popularity as a reliable operation. The PJI rate is higher than other major joints, at over 6% (Kessler et al., 2014). In this study it was suggested that soft-tissue compromise significantly affects the outcome. The soft-tissue reconstruction of defects into the ankle joint can be undertaken using local tissue. Both intrinsic muscle and skin from the dorsum can be used.

References

Adkinson JM, Chung K. Flap reconstruction of the elbow and forearm: a case-based approach. *Hand Clin.* 2014;30:153−63.

Byren I, Bejon P, Atkins BL, et al. One hundred and twelve infected arthroplasties treated with 'DAIR' (debridement, antibiotics and implant retention): antibiotic duration and outcome. *J Antimicrob Chemother.* 2009;63(6):1264−71.

Cetrulo CL, Shiba T, Friel MT, et al. Management of exposed total knee prostheses with microvascular tissue transfer. *Microsurgery.* 2008;28:617−22.

Choa R, Gundle R, Critchely P, Giele H. Successful management of recalcitrant infection related to total hip replacement using pedicled rectus femoris or vastus lateralis muscle flaps. *J Bone Joint Surg (Br).* 2011;93:751−4.

Davami B, Porkhamene G. Versatility of local fasciocutaneous flaps for coverage of soft tissue defects in upper extremity. *J Hand Microsurg.* 2011;3:58−62.

Demirseren ME, Efendioglu K, Demiralp CO, Kilcarslan K, Akkava H. Clinical experience with the reverse-flow anterolateral thigh perforator flap for the reconstruction of soft-tissue defects of the knee and proximal lower leg. *J Plast Reconstr Aesthet Surg.* 2011;64:1613−20.

Gehrke T, Parvizi J. (2013). *Proceedings of the International Consensus meeting on Peri-Prosthetic Joint Infection.* https://www.efort.org/wp-content/uploads/2013/10/Philadelphia_Consensus.pdf

Karki D, Singh AK. The distally-based island ulnar artery perforator flap for wrist defects. *Indian J Plast Surg.* 2007;40:12−17.

Kessler B, Knupp M, Graber P, et al. The treatment and outcome of peri-prosthetic infection of the ankle: a single cohort-centre experience of 34 cases. *Bone Joint J.* 2014;96:772−7.

Laing H, Hancock K, Harrison DH. The exposed total knee replacement prosthesis: a new classification and treatment algorithm. *Br J Plast Surg.* 1992;45(1):66−9.

Mitsala G, Varey AH, O'Neill JK, Chapman TW, Khan U. The distally pedicled gracilis flap for salvage of complex knee wounds. *Injury.* 2014;45:1776−81.

Panni AS, Vasso M, Cerciello Simone Salgarello M. Wound complications in total knee arthroplasty. Which flap is to be used? With or without retention of prosthesis? *Knee Surgery, Sports Traumatology, Arthroscopy.* 2010;19:1060−8.

Rees-Lee JE, Khan U. Superior medial genicular artery (SMGA): a recipient vessel for free flap reconstruction of anterior and medial knee defects. *J Plast Reconstr Aesthetic Surg.* 2011;64:1727−9.

Tiengo C, Macchi V, Porzionato A, et al. Knee region coverage with reversed gracilis pedicle flap (GReSP flap). *JBJS Essent Surg Tech.* 2011;15:1.

Wiedner M, Koch H, Scharnagl E. The superior lateral genicular artery flap for soft-tissue reconstruction around the knee: clinical experience and review of the literature. *Ann Plast Surg.* 2011;66:388−92.

Chapter 7

Specific microbiology issues relating to prosthetic joint infection

'Antibiotics may turn a third rate surgeon into a second rate one; but first rate surgeons don't need them in the first place'

Anon.

Antibiotic prophylaxis: basic rules and evidence

When he was working with Sir Ashley Miles at the Lister Institute in London, John Burke (an American surgeon) established the concept of the 'critical period of implantation'. He used animal models of deliberate challenge with bacteria with a variety of timings for antibiotic administration. His experimental methods and data were definitive: antibiotics would prevent infection, *but only if they were administered in a very clearly defined time window*. He went on to demonstrate that the adverse, purulent consequences of bacterial inoculation were no different from the control group if antibiotics were administered some 4 or more hours after bacterial inoculation. His seminal work was to be proven in a later publication, demonstrating the futility of 'late' antibiotic administration—defined as 4 hours or more after the procedure (Burke, 1984). More recent data demonstrate that a meta-analysis of 26 other meta-analysis studies strongly supported the hypothesis that antibiotic prophylaxis was an effective intervention for preventing surgical site infection over a broad range of surgical procedures. Furthermore, it is now established beyond reasonable doubt that there is never good reason to continue prophylaxis beyond the operative period itself for elective, clean orthopaedic surgery. The situation is far from clear as concerns how long to continue antibiotics postoperatively when dealing with the infected prosthetic joint. Here, success rates depend not on antibiotics but on physical eradication of the organism at the time of surgery through excellent surgical technique and meticulous attention to various issues, such as exhaustive high-volume pulsed lavage and recognition and excision of all tissue considered actually or probably involved in the infective process.

Elective joint replacement in the uninfected case

Many trials have confirmed the efficacy of (appropriately timed) antibiotics for the significant reduction of postoperative infection, both superficial and deep, in the context of elective joint replacement—and indeed this is now considered mandatory, with clear consequences for those who fail to administer such prophylactic antibiotics both in the courts and for the way the quality of their practice is viewed by their managers, peers, and the General Medical Council.

This is perfectly summarized in the latest, revised (2014) Scottish Intercollegiate Network Guidelines (SIGN)—available at www.sign.ac.uk. These guidelines, generated subsequent to very rigorous literature review and subsequent analysis for quality of evidence, should currently be considered as representing the best quality, independent, peer-reviewed standards available.

The duration of antibiotic prophylaxis in relation to outcome has been exhaustively and rigorously investigated in countless studies. The evidence for any and all surgery is clear: there must be adequate concentrations of appropriate antibiotic in those tissues being operated on at the time of operation. There is no evidence that continuing antibiotics beyond this point delivers additional benefit; on the contrary, much evidence exists to show that prolonged antibiotic therapy is not only ineffective, but leads to unintended consequences, relating to generation of both antibiotic resistance and issues related to 'dysbiosis' and diarrhea, whether or not associated with *Clostridium difficile*. There is only one exception, namely operations lasting more than 4 h, or those where there is very significant loss of blood (and therefore antibiotic). In such cases a second dose of prophylaxis is necessary to maintain adequate tissue concentrations within the operative field. Such procedures are relatively uncommon in orthopaedic surgery.

As concerns specific antibiotic choice, this is relatively straightforward and relates to choosing agents with predictable activity against (mostly responsible) Gram-positive organisms (coagulase-negative staphylococci, *Staphylococcus aureus*, streptococci), and (occasionally) Gram-negative organisms (such as *Klebsiella, Enterobacter, Acinetobacter* spp.), administered to provide sufficient tissue levels at or shortly after the time of knife to skin (KTS) to prevent 'critical implantation'.

Suitable choices here (depending on local knowledge and preference) might include a single dose of cefuroxime 1.5 g, or co-amoxiclavulanic acid (Augmentin), together with gentamicin dosed at 1.5 mg/kg, with substitution of teicoplanin dosed at 10 mg/kg for the penicillin-allergic, given in the hour before KTS. Vancomycin or teicoplanin should be used if methicillin-resistant *Staphylococcus aureus* (MRSA) carriage is proven or was proven within a prior 6-month window. Preoperative screening for MRSA remains mandatory for elective implant surgery. Elective surgery should *not* be undertaken under any circumstance if MRSA status is either positive or not determined at the time of the procedure. Subsequent MRSA infection in cases where preoperative screening has not been undertaken represents avoidable harm and prompts likely duty of candour procedure and potential medicolegal challenge. The current MRSA carriage rate in the UK is approximately 2–3%.

Choice of 'prophylaxis/treatment' in the infected, or presumed infected, case

The choice of antibiotic at the time of surgery for prosthetic joint infection (PJI) (not technically 'prophylaxis' but rather 'empiric/adjunctive treatment') for eradication of established infection *must* be driven either by evidence adduced from prior sampling with subsequent isolation and sensitivity testing of the relevant organism or be based on 'best guess' criteria. The specific choice should always be taken in association with the local microbiologist and be driven by prior knowledge of the causative organism and its sensitivity, when known.

In the case of surgery for the proven or presumed infected prosthesis, where an organism has yet to be isolated, the counsel of perfection is to proceed with operation and obtain multiple specimens for culture first and foremost. Such a strategy is acceptable as long as antibiotics are administered within 1, and at the most 2, hours after KTS. If the history leading to a diagnosis of PJI is several weeks, a subsequent diagnosis of coagulase-negative staphylococcal infection is more likely. This mandates use of a glycopeptide (vancomycin or teicoplanin) at the time, as coagulase-negative staphylococcal infection is more likely than not to be resistant to all currently available penicillin and cephalosporin drugs. A single dose of gentamicin should also be given.

There is no clear evidence to mandate with certainty how long such antibiotics should continue, and each case differs and should be approached on its own particular features. It is axiomatic that subsequent isolation of a causative organism should be communicated to the orthopaedic team as soon as it is available, with resolution of such broad-spectrum, 'blind' antibiotic therapy according to findings.

It is equally axiomatic that such decisions should be taken with a fully briefed and engaged microbiologist as part of the team.

A suggested, simple framework for a safe practice

1. Adhere to SIGN guidelines for antibiotic prophylaxis (2014).
2. Decide whether you, or your anaesthetist, is in charge of prescription (whether written or electronic) and administration of antibiotics at anaesthetic induction. Are you clear on this? If not, make it so—and include it in your World Health Organization preoperative checklist. You, the surgeon, are vicariously liable.
3. Choice of antibiotic is secondary—as most antibiotics with which orthopaedic surgeons are familiar continue to be adequate in most situations.
4. Decide whether this is a primary, relatively antibiotic-naïve case, or a secondary, 're-do/known/unknown presumed infection' case. This determines whether choice of antibiotic prophylaxis is standard and protocol-driven or, in the alternative situation, a decision that must be taken with your local microbiologist—this based on available evidence to date—or 'best guess'.
5. Current UK microbial resistance patterns prompt the use of a large, single dose of cefuroxime or co-amoxiclavulanic acid (Augmentin) at KTS. Some trusts have banned cephalosporins because of vancomycin-resistant enterococci, *C. difficile*, or both. Alternatives here include co-amoxiclavulanic acid (Augmentin). For those who have anaphylaxis to penicillins, a combination of a glycopeptide (teicoplanin or vancomycin) and gentamicin is acceptable.

6. The use of adjunctive gentamicin for anything but 'single-dose' blind prophylaxis is questionable. This drug has poor tissue penetration and is toxic, causing renal and vestibular toxicity, the latter leading to deafness and instability. The average orthopaedic case mix is elderly; many are already hard of hearing and/or unstable when standing. Gentamicin will add to these existing challenges to a normal life, sometimes (and unpredictably) irreversibly. This damage is avoidable: a simple rule here is always to avoid gentamicin in those over 60 over and above a single dose for prophylaxis.

Antibiotic use in prosthetic joint infection in the age of resistance

The antibiotics that we use, and are used to using, are becoming increasingly ineffective and precious as resistance emerges, and they must be preserved at all costs. Antibiotic resistance is a global problem and we all have a responsibility for their judicious use.

The cornerstones of such judicious, intelligent, informed, and appropriate use are:

a. *Prophylaxis*—as determined by local guidelines, limited to one or, at the most, two doses for long operations with significant blood loss.

b. *Treatment*—as determined not by guesswork, but by evidence-based, targeted therapy, as determined by isolation of causative organism, their sensitivity pattern, and issues of pharmacokinetic/pharmacodynamic as these apply to specific situations.

c. *Mandatory* multidisciplinary team (MDT) discussion with local microbiologists with specific expertise in orthopaedic infection.

d. As and when necessary, long-term antibiotic deployment, whether oral or via outpatient antibiotic therapy (OPAT), *always* in the context of MDT-driven consensus and downstream planning and consistent review.

e. OPAT is an increasingly necessary option to deploy as in many cases the option for oral antibiotics has disappeared for want of oral antibiotics to which the organism is sensitive.

f. By definition, OPAT involves antibiotics needing intravenous access; it should never be forgotten that this of itself brings risks of contamination, local infection, and bacteraemia. These risks have to be taken in the absence of effective oral therapy.

Background on rising antibiotic resistance

It is every prescribing doctor's responsibility to use antibiotics judiciously. Most have not, considering these precious drugs to be effective forever. They are not—and almost all have been squandered, as resistance becomes anything but futile.

Countless documents have been produced outlining this clear and present threat, and the interested reader is invited to avail themselves of the European Centre for Disease Prevention and Control website, with this 'go-to' URL (https://ecdc. europa.eu/en/home.

Within possibly as little as 2 years, orthopaedic surgeons will be faced with PJI caused by organisms with unpredicted and highly significant resistance profiles, including to 'last-resort' antibiotics such as meropenem.

Alternatives (sometimes very unusual) currently continue to offer possible options; and such options can be made available to patients by treating orthopaedic surgeons within an MDT structure involving microbiologists.

Approach to one- and two-stage surgical management

The evidence for what constitutes 'appropriate' antibiotic therapy in relation to either one- or two-stage surgery is at best poor. There are clear proponents of both strategies. What is also clear is that to insert a new prosthesis in the presence of an inadequately debrided and sterilized operative field is to invite, if not guarantee, relapse and a much worse outcome.

On the other hand, a single-stage procedure, if successful, results in a better, lower risk outcome for the patient over and above avoidance of a second operation.

This remains a hotly debated topic. These issues are discussed in Wongworawat's 'faceoff' debate (Wongworawat, 2013), and the interested reader is invited to follow up on its references for either side of the argument.

What seems clear is that those proponents of single-stage procedures have generated outcomes very similar to those who believe that two stages are necessary. This likely relates more to those centres' very considerable experience and enormous caseload; it is likely that those factors of 'experience' contribute to their excellent outcomes just as much as issues of bacteria and their treatment. Notably, microbiologists feature centrally in such units; such close collaboration doubtless enhances outcomes.

In the absence of definitive data, we currently do not know how long to continue antibiotic therapy after either a debridement, antibiotic and implant retention (DAIR) procedure, or after implant replacement in the treatment of PJI.

It is, however, clear that in principle no amount of antibiotic administered in the context of infection proven to involve a prosthesis where biofilm is present will result in bacteriological 'cure'.

Despite continuing and misguided overreliance by some orthopaedic surgeons on the perceived magical powers of antibiotics, this argument is absolute. This author's experience is of some 20 years' observation of the eventual futility of antibiotics in cases where there is evidence of bacterial contact, colonization, and biofilm formation on the surface of a prosthetic joint. In the absence of a scenario where reoperation presents a danger to life, or is refused by the patient, the best that can be hoped for is partial control of the infection, with no hope of eventual 'cure'.

Outpatient antibiotic therapy

OPAT continues to become more and more prominent in clinical care pathways and individual hospital portfolios. The main drivers for this expansion in both volume and indications are: a) the pressure to maximize inpatient bed usage and shorten lengths of stay; and b) the decreasingly effective armamentarium of orally available antibiotics in the age of ever-increasing antibiotic resistance.

The critical elements of a safe and efficient service include:

1. A single pathway for referrals and entry into the OPAT programme.

2. Patients considered for OPAT must have been assessed and approved for suitability by a clinical microbiologist to minimize inappropriate or ineffective antibiotic use.

3. There must be a prompt, efficient, and safe line insertion service.

4. There must be clear governance procedures around line care, together with a set of inclusion/exclusion criteria for bringing into service.

5. There must be a regular review in a clinic of the line by a specialist nurse. In addition, there must be responsive, same-day access to a clinical nurse specialist/doctor to deal with any complications that may arise (line blockage, infection).

6. There must be input from an infection doctor—ideally a consultant—this is because heavily protocol-driven care often leads to inflexibility in an area of considerable complexity, and unnecessary and inappropriate rule-driven exclusion.

7. There must be regular medical review of any and all clinical problems and antibiotic choice—to ensure prompt diagnosis of intravenous thoracic outlet syndromes and issues of possible escalation when failing.

8. There must be a clearly articulated policy of administration of antibiotics after discharge if this is considered acceptable and appropriate. This policy should provide evidence relating to how antibiotics are given and by whom.

9. There must be virtual MDT ward rounds—at least weekly—at which senior orthopaedic doctors should be in attendance to discuss their complex patients.

10. There must be an electronic patient record, accessible by all members of the patients' MDT.

There must *not* be:

1. Multiple referral pathways into service.

2. No central oversight of who is on OPAT in the community.

3. A poorly standardized, slow, or unpredictable line insertion service.

4. No centrally held accessible record of the patient once discharged.

5. No infectious diseases/microbiology input into choice and duration of antibiotic.

You can find a document which sets out the basis and structures for an OPAT service here: http://bsac.org.uk/wp-content/uploads/2014/03/BSAC-BPAIIG-p-OPAT-good-practice-recommendations_for-consultation.pdf.

Outpatient antibiotic therapy: when to use it

Whilst little well-defined, objective data exist concerning duration of antibiotic treatment in the various scenarios of post-PJI management, most, if not almost all, surgeons will opt for a 'safe' (if not necessary) extended treatment period.

Many PJIs now involve organisms that have acquired extended resistance to many orally available antibiotics—in some cases all.

There is no evidence that, if oral alternatives are available, these will not be equally efficacious as intravenous alternatives if they have suitable pharmacokinetic/pharmacodynamic characteristics.

In addition, therapy constructed around and needing intravenous administration by definition implies insertion of a long line, usually a peripherally inserted central catheter (PICC) line, for the duration of therapy. This is not without risk of iatrogenic line-associated bacteraemia.

The advantages for the patient when a long inpatient stay is the only alternative are clear. Is it also possible in some circumstances to teach the patients to administer their own antibiotics if appropriate and possible.

Monitoring/stopping rules

There are no evidence-based and universally applicable rules. Each and every case should be discussed in a multidisciplinary context, as no two cases are likely to be identical with regard to risk/benefit ratios, treatment options, etc.

The basic universal premises that do apply, however, are:

a. Judicious, regular, close follow-up.

b. Careful documentation and description of clinical features of infection and its resolution, such as swelling, erythema, fever, pain, and functionality.

c. Monitoring of blood parameters: C-reactive protein, white blood cells, and development or reversal of anaemia of chronic infection as a surrogate of relapse or cure.

d. A keen eye for when progress ceases in the face of appropriate antibiotics, prompting a low threshold for reconsideration of the need for diagnostics and more options, almost always related to the need for further surgery rather than a change in antibiotics. The latter invariably fails.

The particular problem of Pseudomonas and Candida in prosthetic joint infection

P. aeruginosa and *C. albicans* stand out as particularly recalcitrant infections. This is because of these organisms' particular ability to develop and survive within their own biofilm over and above most other organisms. If it is not possible to entirely physically 'clean' prostheses contaminated with these organisms, then antibiotic/antifungal therapy should only be used for purposes of suppression where removal (and a subsequent downstream plan for replacement) is either inappropriate, un-acceptably high risk, or declined as an option by the patient.

In such cases, the impossibility of cure (as opposed to, at best, long-term suppression) should be made quite clear to the patient. The decision in this situation is quite clear: a) surgical removal of the implant and start again (as a two-stage procedure) or lifelong suppression, with the clear and present risk of antibiotic suppression failure secondary to overgrowth and replacement by a resistant clone. It is imperative to ensure that the patient is presented with these options and allowed to consider them when apprised, so that they may be involved in these difficult decisions and remain in charge of their fate. In addition, long-term, low levels of systemic inflammation are now known to shorten life through several mechanisms, such as amyloid deposition and renal failure and atherosclerosis to name but two. Surgeons should make those patients who have the choice to undergo curative surgery, as opposed to living with chronic infection, aware of the consequences of their decision.

Myths and facts about what 'immunosuppression' actually means in practice

Individual factors: how to define and approach the concept of 'immunosuppression'—and how this should change your practice.

Little data exist to inform this increasingly important matter. 'Immunosuppression' may be due to disease, the consequences of its treatment, or both. Outcomes for patients with rheumatoid arthritis are worse (Hsieh et al., 2013)—whether this relates to the disease process itself, the underlying damage to tissues, the drugs used for control, or a combination of these factors is not known.

And yet this crude and inappropriate word is used liberally, inappropriately, and with little, if any, evidence-based justification.

Host control of bacteria and fungi relies on recognition/opsonization and phagocytosis by functional polymorphs. In theory, any process that degrades any part of this pathway will increase susceptibility to, and outcome of, bacterial infection. Diabetes is also a proven factor increasing risk, probably through both higher tissue glucose levels as well as well-described effects on immune cell recognition of pathogens.

There is little high-quality evidence to define 'immunosuppression' properly. Probably more important is an objective assessment of individual patients' collated comorbidities (diabetes, age, targeted immunosuppressive therapy, steroids, to name but a few). This plays in to the emerging theme of 'precision medicine', i.e. wrapping tailor-made therapy and management according to the individual.

Such an approach will likely be the next driver toward better outcomes for patients and should be endorsed by all surgeons undertaking this work.

Methicillin-resistant *Staphylococcus aureus*

This organism's UK prevalence has tumbled over the past 7 years subsequent to the government's highly effective campaign of control. It continues to circulate, however, in the community—especially in nursing homes. Screening for MRSA carriage, preferably done by same-day molecular technology, remains mandatory for most orthopaedic procedures, and all involving implants other than K-wires. 'Decontamination' involves head-to-toe exposure over a 5-day period to either chlorhexidine or biguanide antiseptic solutions and shampoo, together with application of either chlorhexidine or mupirocin cream into the nostrils. This is not always successful—often because patients do not strictly adhere to the application process. Even if not successful, however, these decolonization regimens result in very significant (several log order) drops in MRSA skin colonization. Many hip implants are performed as an emergency after falls; in this scenario, especially if the patient comes from a nursing home, it would be prudent to assume MRSA colonization whilst waiting for the result and attempt at least one round of chlorhexidine application before surgery, together with appropriate antibiotic prophylaxis with a glycopeptide.

Conclusions

Ten suggested 'dos and don'ts'

Do:

a. Always involve your local microbiologists.

b. Always attempt to isolate the causative organism, without which no evidence-based and rational therapy plan can be constructed.

c. Consider the rationale for your and your patients' decisions concerning one- as opposed to two-stage replacement.

d. Treat local, superficial postoperative infections very aggressively with local debridement and lavage before the organisms gain access to the implant.

e. Always send too many intraoperative deep specimens, rather than not enough.

f. Consider as many 're-looks' as might be necessary when attempting to eradicate early, deep infection.

Do *not*:

a. Rely on antibiotics only, if you believe that metalwork is involved; this is bound to fail.

b. Treat all postoperative infections empirically and automatically with anti-staphylococcal agents, such as flucloxacillin, *without* sending at least one specimen deeper than the edges of the wound. Many such infections are not due to these organisms, and, indeed, may be made worse by them.

c. Stitch gaping wounds, thereby 'sealing in' organisms whose direction of travel will then be to deeper tissues and the implant.

d. Neglect to follow up on all microbiology results in a timely fashion with a microbiology colleague. The findings might vary from irrelevant to central to your case and your patient's outcome.

References

Burke JF. Ashley A. Miles and the prevention of infection following surgery. *Arch Surg.* 1984;119(1):17–19.

Hsieh PH, Huang KC, Shih HN. Prosthetic joint infection in patients with rheumatoid arthritis: an out-come analysis compared with controls. *PLoS One.* 2013;8(8):e71666.

Wongworawat MD. Clinical faceoff: one- versus two-stage exchange arthroplasty for prosthetic joint infections. *Clin Orthop Relat Res.* 2013;471(6):1750–3.

Chapter 8

Revision arthroplasty networks

Revision arthroplasty surgery demand is increasing in the UK. The causes of this are multifactorial but include an aging population, an increased number of primary procedures, and many other factors, including implant design, surgical technique, and infection (Kurtz et al., 2007a; b; 2008). Outcomes are worst for revision total knee replacement (TKR), with greater rate and complexity of complications and the need for further surgery. A strategy is needed for classifying the complexity of revision surgery such that the best revision is performed at the earliest opportunity by the most appropriate surgeon, all to the patient's benefit.

There has been much recent focus on total joint replacement and revision surgery, particularly in England and Wales, with the publication of the Getting it Right First Time (GiRFT) report (Briggs, 2015). Within the GiRFT report is a strong recommendation that a revision network strategy should be established around the country to optimize the outcome from revision arthroplasty surgery and minimize the cost of its delivery. Patient complications and morbidity are increased and outcomes worsened when comparing low-volume with high-volume centres undertaking revision arthroplasty (Katz et al., 2001; Feinglass et al., 2004; Cram et al., 2007; Pulido et al., 2008; Marlow et al., 2010).

Proposed model for revision networks

It has been proposed that revision networks are established around the country and operate on a hub-and-spoke model. A number of hospitals should therefore work *together* to develop this system. A large hospital, which performs the majority of revision surgery in that area, should act as the operational centre for the revision network. All revision cases should be presented to the network both from the hub-and-spoke hospitals. All revision cases should be discussed by all participating personnel and an action plan developed and recorded, with complex cases being transferred to the larger central hospital.

Proposed operating framework

The frequency of meetings will depend on the volume of revisions done in the region, but a weekly meeting would be ideal. This could be face to face but is more reliably delivered with video conferencing and integrated imaging facilities (such as Picture Archiving and Communications System) to allow all images to be viewed.

Out of these meetings urgent ad hoc telephone contact with named revision surgeons for emergency patients should be available.

The service should be run by a network coordinator who will work with all of the sites participating to collate the information and records for discussion. The host site will provide a multidisciplinary team to include revision surgical specialists, specialist microbiologist, a network coordinator, and other surgical specialities as indicated by the information provided to include plastic surgical attendees and vascular surgical expertise, if required. A specific musculoskeletal radiologist should also be on hand to advise on specialist imaging, and physiotherapy and occupational therapy expertise should also be available, if required.

It should be mandated that all revision procedures, all infected joint replacements, and all complex primary procedures be discussed.

The contents of the discussion from the video conference should be recorded for governance purposes and this record, together with a treatment plan, should be circulated to all and shared with the patient and filed in the notes. This should be signed by the chair of the meeting who may be based at the central location. This model has been poneered in the East Midlands to good effect (Bloch et al., 2017).

Aims of the revision network

The aim of the process is to allow discussion to occur of all complex revision cases and for a surgical plan to be agreed. The identification of those patients likely to have perioperative complications and potentially worse outcomes can lead to decisions on where, how, and who performs the revision TKR, to the patient's benefit. To understand the specialization needed in managing revision TKR the surgeon must appreciate multiple principles, i.e. extensile approaches, bone reconstruction, joint line and balance, and optimizing fixation. To undertake revision TKR the surgeon must be able to identify the cause of failure, the complexity of individual cases, and have the relevant experience, equipment, and multidisciplinary backup before embarking on what is demanding surgery.

The aim of the process is to allow discussion to occur of all complex revision cases and for a surgical plan to be identified.

Within the hub-and-spoke environment the use of loan kit should be reduced to a minimum, which may require transfer of patients into the central hub for specialist revision surgery. The reduction in use of loan kits has significant potential to reduce cost for the management of these complex patients (Briggs, 2015).

Audit of the revision network is important to ensure that the plans generated are accurate. The audit should include how often deviation from the plan occurs and the reasons that this deviation occurred. Clinical audit to review the outcome of the intervention should also be regularly performed, with suggested 6-monthly face-to-face meetings of the revision network members to discuss cases and further improve their outcomes.

National Joint Registry is mandatory and requires careful and completed entry.

References

Bloch B, Raglan M, Manktelow A, James P. The East Midlands Specilaist Orthopaedic Network: the future of revision arthroplasty? RCS Bulletin 2017;99(2):66–70.

Briggs T. A national review of adult elective orthopaedic services in England. Getting it right first time. March 2015, http://gettingitrightfirsttime.co.uk/.

Cram P, Vaughan-Sarrazin MS, Wolf B, Katz JN, Rosenthal GE. A comparison of total hip and knee replacement in specialty and general hospitals. *J Bone Joint Surg Am.* 2007;89(8):1675–84.

Feinglass J, Koo S, Koh J. Revision total knee arthroplasty complication rates in Northern Illinois. *Clin Orthop Relat Res.* 2004;429:279–85.

Katz JN, Losina E, Barrett J, et al. Association between hospital and surgeon procedure volume and outcomes of total hip replacement in the United States medicare population. *J Bone Joint Surg Am.* 2001;83-A(11):1622–9.

Kurtz SM, Ong KL, Schmier S, et al. Future clinical and economic impact of revision total hip and knee arthroplasty. *J Bone Joint Surg Am.* 2007a;89:144–51.

Kurtz S, Ong K, Lau E, Mowat F, Halpern M. Projections of primary and revision hip and knee arthroplasty in the United States from 2005 to 2030. *J Bone Joint Surg Am.* 2007b;89(4):780–5.

Kurtz SM, Lau E, Schmier J, Ong KL, Zhao K, Parvizi J. Infection burden for hip and knee arthroplasty in the United States. *J Arthroplasty.* 2008;23(7):984–91.

Marlow NE, Barraclough B, Collier NA, et al. Centralization and the relationship between volume and outcome in knee arthroplasty procedures. *ANZ J Surg.* 2010;80(4):234–41.

Pulido L, Parvizi J, Macgibany M, et al. In hospital complications after total joint arthroplasty. *J Arthroplasty.* 2008;23(6: Suppl. 1):139–45.

Chapter 9

Case histories

Introduction

This chapter provides several typical cases encountered in patients who develop infection in prosthetic joints after surgery. The impact on the patient is immense and the surgical options are challenging; prevention and reducing the incidence is the key to addressing this problem. The following clinical cases reflect on the typical presentation of established and latent infections. Both the assessment and the definitive management will be considered, as well as the microbiology profiles and the need for protracted antibiotics.

Case 1—flap selection

This case illustrates extracapsular infection in a limited area and how this can be managed with the use of excision and local skin flap transfer. The case is of an elderly man who underwent a total knee arthroplasty. Several weeks later the surgical incision developed small pustules. His blood markers were low and he underwent a joint aspiration under aseptic theatre conditions, which was also sterile. The patient was taken to theatre jointly by consultant orthopaedic and plastic surgeons. The sinuses were excised and a decision reached that this was extracapsular. Owing to the location and small size of the wound a decision was made to utilize the laxity of the skin on the medial aspect of the knee and undertake a local random pattern fasciocutaneous flap with a back-cut to aid rotation. The wound healed uneventfully. (See illustrations C1.1 and C1.2).

C1.1

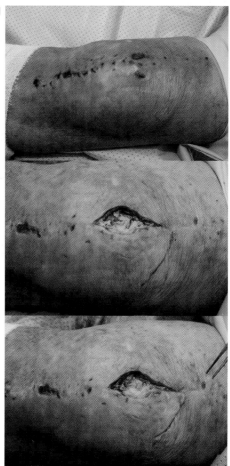

C1.2

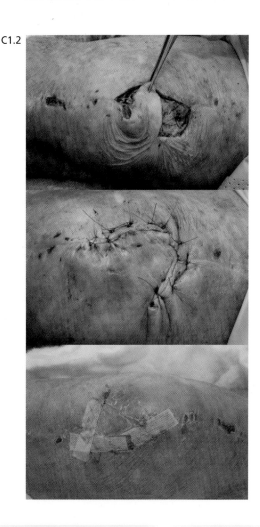

Case 2—difficult wounds around the knee

The use of free tissue transfer around the knee joint can only be successful when due consideration is paid in the planning of such difficult operations. Defects such as the one illustrated in this case show that when local tissue cannot be used then more demanding procedures must be entrained to avoid a high amputation.

The case is of a male patient who had undergone a total knee arthroplasty many years after suffering periarticular trauma. He had several previous skin incisions. He developed a prosthetic joint infection (PJI) and skin necrosis, which, after excision and negative pressure wound therapy, left him with a large defect over the lateral and anterior surfaces of the knee area. A salvage was planned with the use of a large skin flap and the lateral genicular vessels as recipients for the free flap transfer. These vessels are under the fascial condensations and the retinacular fibres laterally. The vessels are of a good size to accept and support free tissue transfer. The limb was salvaged without any adverse events (see Illustrations C2.1–C2.3).

C2.1

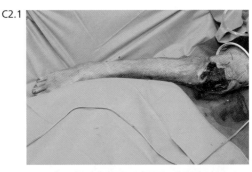

C2.2

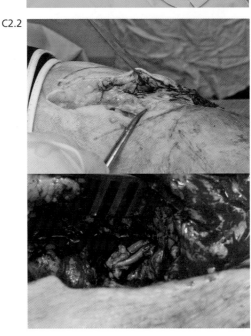

C2.3

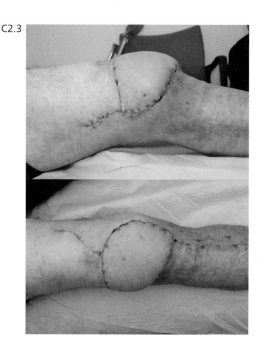

Case 3—ankle joint prosthetic joint infection

This case illustrates that, in high-risk patients, skin necrosis and PJI may coexist. The prospect of limb salvage remains poor in such individuals.

The patient was a young patient with rheumatoid arthritis and vasculitis. She had previously had mid-foot surgery and presented with ankle pain. She underwent a total ankle replacement (Illustration C3.1). However, during that procedure it was noted that the foot was poorly perfused. Vascular reconstruction was undertaken. Subsequent skin necrosis and infection ensued (Illustration C3.2).

To control the infection and have any hope of limb salvage she underwent excision of the necrotic skin and removal of the implant (Illustration C3.3). It was also noted that the circulation of the foot remained poor, rendering limb salvage unpredictable. Ultimately a below-knee amputation was undertaken for this case of PJI.

C3.1

LEFT

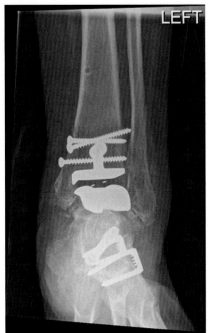

C3.2

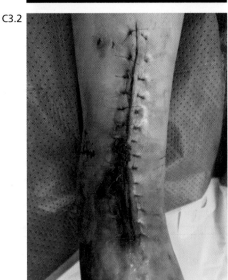

C3.3

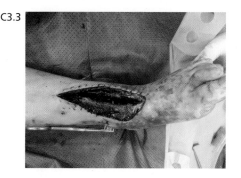

61

Case 4—comprehensive membrane resection and flap

This case illustrates the need for aggressive and comprehensive membrane resection as well as any soft-tissue involvement. The case is of an elderly male who underwent a total knee replacement. He developed a PJI but this was treated by several washouts and antibiotic suppression for several months by the surgeon treating him. He was eventually referred to the Ortho-Plastic centre, having become septic. He had obvious suppuration and loosening of the implant. He did not want an amputation and fusion was thought to be a high-risk procedure. It was then decided to undertake a two-stage salvage.

Stage one was planned for a comprehensive membrane resection with explantation of the entire implant plus a free tissue transfer. Stage one was aided by taking the tibial tuberosity with the extensor mechanism off as one unit for ease of access. Stage two was a revision arthroplasty with a hinge restraint.

See Illustrations C4.1–C4.5.

C4.1

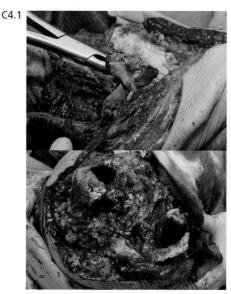

C4.2

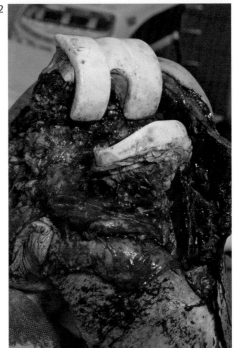

C4.3

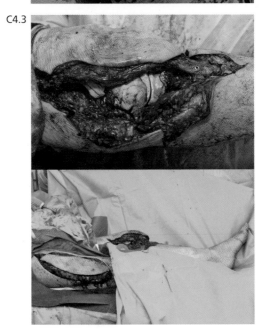

C4.4

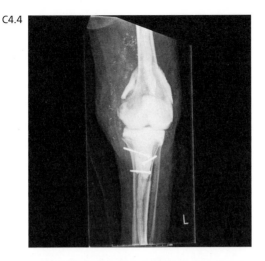

C4.5

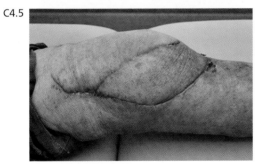

Index

Notes Figures and boxed material are indicated by an italic *f* or *b* following the page number. *vs.* indicates a comparison or differential diagnosis